Clinical risk management

An introductory text
for mental health clinicians

Clinical risk management

An introductory text
for mental health clinicians

Tom Flewett

MB, BS, MRCPsych, FRANZCP, FAChAM
Consultant Psychiatrist/Addiction Specialist
Community Alcohol and Drugs Service
Capital and Coast Health
Wellington, New Zealand

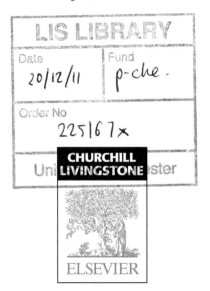

CHURCHILL LIVINGSTONE

ELSEVIER

Sydney   Edinburgh   London   New York
Philadelphia   St Louis   Toronto

Churchill Livingstone
is an imprint of Elsevier

Elsevier Australia. ACN 001 002 357
(a division of Reed International Books Australia Pty Ltd)
Tower 1, 475 Victoria Avenue, Chatswood, NSW 2067

ELSEVIER

© 2010 Elsevier Australia

National Library of Australia Cataloguing-in-Publication Data

---

Flewett, Tom.

Clinical risk management : an introductory text for mental health clinicians / Tom Flewett.

9780729539340 (pbk.)

Includes index.
Bibliography.

Crisis intervention (Mental health services)
Mental health facilities--Risk management.
Psychiatry.

616.89025

Publisher: Sophie Kaliniecki
Developmental Editor: Sabrina Chew/Neli Bryant
Publishing Services Manager: Helena Klijn
Project Coordinators: Lauren Allsop/Karen Griffiths
Edited by Forsyth Publishing Services
Proofread by Tim Learner
Cover and internal design by Lisa Petroff
Index by Forsyth Publishing Services
Typeset by TNQ Books and Journals
Printed by 1010 Printing International Limited

▓ FOREWORD

I was pleased to read this thoughtful book written by clinician Tom Flewett, whose main interests lie outside forensic mental health. Like many other clinicians, Dr Flewett's approach to perceived and actual risk is not based on 'the prediction of dangerousness' but on clear clinical assessment, wise decision-making and adequate systems of accountability.

Risk is ubiquitous. mental health, in its widest dimensions, maps across the whole of life. Assessment therefore entails 'teasing out' capacity and competence issues from the myriad decisions a patient (or service-user) might make on a daily basis; for example, whether to (continue to) take substances, whether to comply with medical advice, how to manage stress, whether to change jobs, and so on.

As Dr Flewett points out, the outcome of a particular risk management strategy does not determine the adequacy of the risk management process. Rather, adequacy is determined by the careful and methodical assessment and implementation of prudent risk management strategies agreed in consultation with the patient and his or her family or supporters.

Some authors have stated that risk management cannot coexist with a 'recovery' focus. For most of us risk management is practised on a daily basis (e.g. safely crossing the road) and because of this we are able to enjoy life to the full. Identifying and managing risk is not just the preserve of the forensic clinician but of every clinician.

The book is well set out and easy to read and is replete with helpful practical suggestions and clinical vignettes covering the whole of mental health and addictions.

I enjoyed reading Dr Flewett's book and commend him for his service to good clinical practice and patient wellbeing.

D G Chaplow (Dr)
QSO, MB, ChB, FRANZCP
Director, Mental Health and Chief Advisor,
Ministry of Health, Wellington NZ

▦ DISCLAIMER

The information contained in this book is intended to assist but not replace the use of sound clinical judgment when assessing and managing risks. The author accepts no responsibility or liability for errors or adverse consequences arising from the use of information contained in this book.

■I CONTENTS

■■ PREFACE

This book started as a brief, one-hour training session on risk for mental health clinicians and has slowly grown over a period of six years. It was partially driven by my increasing awareness that I did not understand the science of risk management and the processes which I had been applying almost intuitively for some years. The introduction of tick-box forms for risk management made me feel that I had been doing something wrong in my clinical practice and I wondered if my training had been deficient.

I found myself observing that the degree of anxiety I felt about risk decision making around suicidal patients was different to that of my colleagues. The processes that I went through to determine suicidality or potential for violence were also substantially different at times. In some respects, I felt fortunate not to be working in the UK where the development of risk assessment and management has been heavily coloured by the events surrounding the death of Johnathan Zito, who was killed in 1992 by Christopher Clunis, a patient suffering from schizophrenia. The subsequent inquiry found a series of missed opportunities to assess risk adequately and plan appropriate care. The trend of risk assessment and management being driven by external agencies and not clinicians was initiated to a large extent by this single event.

My colleagues in the UK have had risk brought into the spotlight by the government and media to a much greater extent than seemed to be the case for those working elsewhere.[1] In New Zealand we have been relatively fortunate in some respects in that our processes for assessing and managing risk have been driven to a greater extent by clinicians, which has afforded us a sense of 'buy-in' which does not seem to be evident in the UK.

The task of deconstructing my clinical practice and exploring that of colleagues has led to many interesting discussions which have been distilled into the structure embedded in this book. Coming full circle and reconstructing my work I am now happily convinced that the essence of risk management is good clinical practice but it should be assisted by as much help as can be had from structured analysis of known risk factors. If risk within the clinical setting is managed well, clinical management

[1]Rethinking risk to others in mental health services. Final report of a scoping group. June 2008. Royal College of Psychiatrists College Report CR 150.

is improved. Better patient care reduces risk for the public. As risk management improves, clinician anxiety lessens substantially, which leads to less defensive practice and more energy being available for the process of good clinical work.

Within the book, the emphasis is on the care of the patient as opposed to protection of the public or clinicians. Whilst recognising that there is a role of public protection within risk management, I have tended towards the stance of saying that good risk management is based on good patient care and this will lead to protection of the public without extra need for custodial care.

A by-product of my exploration of risk has been the developing capacity to take a stand against the use of the concept of risk as the new form of stigma applied to psychiatric patients.[2] There is a view held by some members of the public that risk is an unacceptable danger. We have all seen statements made in the media that there should be no high-risk patients in the community. This is another form of the stigma which caused patients in Victorian times to be locked up in asylums. There has also been a public view that mental health workers should be able to prevent all suicide or all episodes of violence committed by patients with mental illness. Bringing risk assessment and management firmly back into the realm of good clinical practice may help reduce the development of stigma being related to risk.

The literature on risk has grown exponentially in recent years and, for most practitioners, it is difficult to keep up. The majority of the risk literature focuses on the risk for violence, but much of it can be transferred to all the risks which are met within routine clinical practice. Within the book I have utilised the documentation that has been used in my work setting in recent times. It is in keeping with much that is recommended in the risk literature and uses empirically developed risk factors as prompts within a structured form of assessment. This documentation is evolving on a regular basis as a result of feedback received from patients and clinicians. If the format of the documentation within this book works for you, I hope you will feel free to use it, but if your setting, culture or workplace is different, feel free to change the documentation to something which works for you, your patients and their families. Alternatively, use one of the standardised tools available for the assessment and management of risk.

The term 'patient' is used in this book to denote a person who suffers. If you would rather use the term client or service user, you can substitute whichever term feels best for you.

[2]Undrill G 2000 The risks of risk assessment. *Advances in Psychiatric Treatment*, 13:291–7.

Although definitions of risk have been included in the body of this book, the use of the word 'risk' by mental health clinicians does not always agree with dictionary definitions. When asked what the risk is, clinicians will often simply describe the possible adverse outcome rather than discussing the '*likelihood* of the adverse outcome' occurring. In the book, rather than using the phrase 'adverse outcome' or 'harmful behaviour', I have chosen to use the words 'risk behaviour'.

■■ AUTHOR

Doctor Tom Flewett completed his medical training from the London Hospital Medical School in 1980. After completing his psychiatric training in south-west England, he moved to New Zealand in the late 1980s. The next decade was spent as a general adult psychiatrist in Hawke's Bay, North Island, New Zealand. After moving to Wellington, he spent 5 years working with patients with severe borderline personality disorder before moving into his current post as a consultant psychiatrist/addiction specialist where he has worked for the last 8 years.

The management of risk at an individual and systemic level has been a long-term interest. His interest in psychodynamic theory, the years spent caring for patients in acute psychiatric settings and managing the chronic risk associated with severe personality disorder has strongly influenced the practical content of this book. His more recent work in the addiction field has enabled a common component of risk assessment and management to be included in the examples.

▓▌ ACKNOWLEDGEMENTS

Thanks to Capital Coast District Health Board staff, especially Pip Bradley, Ken McDonnell, Andrew Highnet, and the original risk training team of June Robertson, Reg Orovwuje and Alicia Morris for their ideas and energy. Thanks also to Murray Patton and Andy Carroll for supportive criticism along the way and to the other external reviewers. Special thanks to Linda for her thoughtful comments and for tolerating the many hours of absence from home life.

PART 1

INTRODUCTION TO RISK IN MENTAL HEALTH

1 Why focus on risk?

> Clinical risk assessment should be motivated primarily by the intention to provide a patient with better treatment and care.[1]

This book is designed to assist clinical practice by providing the knowledge and skills to apply sound risk management techniques in day-to-day work. The purpose of applying these risk management techniques is to provide better outcomes for patients, staff and the community. The risk management processes contained in this book aim to ensure that all reasonable steps to promote wellbeing and provide adequate safeguards against avoidable harm have been taken during a patient's treatment and care. Understanding and pursuing the assessment (and management) of risk to oneself and others is part of the required standard of ordinary clinical practice.[2] This book is primarily a clinical guide, but can also be used as a teaching tool.

Principles of risk management

Within mental health settings, risk management used to be considered the business of predicting and preventing dangerousness.

> The traditional focus of risk-taking, in mental disorder services, involved concentrating on a patient's dangerousness. With this approach, there was an implicit assumption that 'risk' was limited to failures, to the causing of harm.[3]

The focus of risk management today is not so much on the end point of preventing the adverse outcome, but more on enhancing clinicians' performance at all stages of treatment to achieve a good outcome for the patient. This is attained through focus on:

- skills acquisition and decision-making
- management of risk factors in the context of illness and with recovery principles in mind
- team work
- organisational factors.

> Much medical effort goes into managing the risks of complications of disease processes rather than managing the symptoms of the disease itself. Hypertension is the classic example, with no symptoms but plenty of treatments, all aiming to reduce the risk of complications such as strokes and myocardial infarctions. Psychiatry's misfortune has been to choose diseases where the complications ... are homicide, suicide or reduced capacity for self-care and vulnerability.[4]

This problem becomes the nub of risk management within mental health. On the one hand clinicians try to treat the illness while at the same time managing the risk, which is often a complication of the disease process rather than a symptom of the disease itself. 'Risk, especially violence, can be a preventable complication of some types of mental disorder.'[5]

This book focuses primarily on skills acquisition and the process of decision-making. It provides opportunities to practise some of the suggested techniques in the case examples. Organisational factors are touched on briefly but are predominantly the brief of senior clinicians, team leaders and clinical leaders. Detailed discussion of organisational factors is beyond the scope of this book but an introduction is given in Part 4.

Guidelines vary from country to country and are dependent mostly on the structure of health services rather than clinical differences. Good risk management involves having knowledge of guidelines and knowing how to access them. Guidelines should be available in printed form at your workplace. Some guidelines currently available, and useful in conjunction with this book, include:

Suicide
- New Zealand Suicide Guidelines 2003. Available from www.nzgg.org.nz
  - Click on 'Publications' and then 'Mental Health'.

Risk to others
- Guidelines for the Assessment and Management of Risk to Others, 2006. Available from www.tepou.co.nz/page/tepou_23.php
  - Click on 'Publications'.
- Violence: The short-term management of disturbed/violent behaviour in inpatient psychiatric settings and Emergency Departments (EDs). Available from National Institute of Clinical Excellence: http://www.nice.org.uk/Guidance/CG/Published

Self-harm
- Australasian Self-harm Guidelines. Summary in *Australasian Psychiatry*, 2003 (11)2: 150–5.
- Guidelines for the Management of Deliberate Self-harm in Young People. Available from Australasian College of Emergency Medicine and Royal Australian and New Zealand College of Psychiatrists.
- Self-harm: The Short-Term Physical and Psychological Management and Secondary Prevention of Self-harm in Primary and Secondary Care. Available from National Institute of Clinical Excellence: http://www.nice.org.uk/Guidance/CG/Published

This book is only one step in learning about risk assessment and management. Further steps include:
- Implementing the clinical skills learned and gaining familiarity with the process of risk assessment and management. Being unfamiliar with a task can increase the likelihood of error by a factor of 17.[6]
- Team and individual support through team meetings, seeking advice from a senior colleague, supervision, audits, reviews, second opinions, etc.

The book is divided into four parts. The first part, introduction to risk in mental health, is a necessary prerequisite for the second part, clinical skills training. Part 3 focuses on risk factors for suicide, self-harm and violence, and part 4 covers areas which are primarily the concern of advanced practitioners although all clinicians need some knowledge of these areas.

The development of a risk culture within mental health services

It is not possible to practise any branch of medicine free from risk and uncertainty.[7]

All mental health clinicians should be trained in the assessment and management of suicidality and violence. There is a growing body of evidence to assist the clinician in making more structured decisions in his/her assessment and management of risk. In more recent times, risk management has been introduced as a phrase to encapsulate much of what clinicians have always done in a relatively unstructured way.

In the 1960s insurance companies in the United States coined the phrase 'risk management'[8] and around the same time an increasing number of medical lawsuits led to insurance companies applying the same concepts to the health sector.[9] Over the last 50 years there has been a movement towards greater accountability for all professionals and a parallel movement of consumer empowerment. Litigation and complaints have continued to become an ever-present component of clinical practice whilst the *culture of blame* in which we live has become more pronounced.[10]

Political focus and media commentary on (risk) have increased. Society has become, in general, more risk averse.[11] Across all media, people with a mental disorder are portrayed in a negative manner, and typically as dangerous.[12] The pendulum may be swinging, however, with calls for the culture of blame to be given up.[13] Some clinicians feel that they work in a riskier environment but it may be that this is a response to increased scrutiny and accountability of their work. Consumer empowerment and access to information has allowed patients to become more aware of treatment options and more able to demand the best quality of care available. This change should be welcomed. Clinicians have had to adapt to this new environment: some have been more successful than others. Some clinicians may be more defensive in their practice as a result of anxiety driven by a fear of accountability and a fear of complaints being laid against them. 'The effects of this (blame) culture appear to be counterproductive, leading to defensive practice, and undermining both professional morale and recruitment into the profession.'[14]

Clinicians may think they are in the vicious circle outlined in Figure 1.1.[15]

The blame culture is unlikely to change in the near future. Clinicians are increasingly accountable, which is appropriate, but if increased

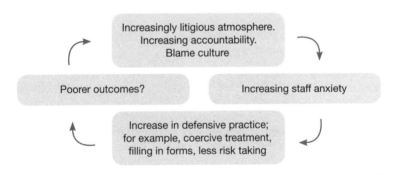

Figure 1.1 Potential consequences of the blame culture on risk management

accountability is allowed to heighten anxiety, clinical practice will be stifled.

> The danger of frequent legislative changes, and a growing emphasis on blame attribution when things go wrong, is that professionals can feel that they lack expertise in implementing unfamiliar procedures or using new terminology. It is important to remember that the basic standards of good clinical practice have changed very little and adherence to them will avoid most pitfalls.[16]

Out of concern about the 'blame culture', Carson (2008)[17] developed proposals which were to be understood as an integrated program for tackling blame culture. The evidence and theory to support these proposals were presented in a recent book by Carson and Bain (2008).[18]

The House of Lords, in a leading court case on the standard of care expected of professionals, assumed that 'risk' involved the chance of harm and it specifically recognised that it would be appropriate to balance this with the chances of benefit (*Bolitho v City and Hackney Health Authority* [1998] AC 232). Risk decisions need to be made with clear thought given to the potential benefits. These benefits need to be articulated within the decision-making process.

Carson's proposals for tackling the blame culture are outlined below. He says they are self-evident 'truths' about risk-taking, and are generally agreed with by professional associations and employers. As this should improve staff morale, and reduce the risk of litigation, employers ought to embrace these principles.[19]

- Risk is part of life so by definition, it is inevitable that harm will sometimes occur, irrespective of the quality of risk decisions and risk management.
- The quality of a risk decision cannot properly be impugned just because harm resulted. Equally a risk decision should not be assumed good just because no harm occurred. And failure to make any necessary decision may be the cause of harm, and deserves censure.
- When judging a risk decision, both the risk assessment and risk management should be considered, including the quantity and quality of resources made available for the latter.
- By definition, risk assessment involves imperfect knowledge and risk management involves finite resources.
- Risk assessment inevitably involves difficult decisions about values. That others would have made different decisions does not, on its own, indicate that a poor or improper decision was made.

- Anyone, including managers, supervisors, systems designers and employers (i.e. not only those in the front line) can be the cause of poor risk decision-making, such as where insufficient or inappropriate support, advice, information, training or other resources are provided.
- If risk-taking is to improve then there must be an analysis of good decision-making, not just inquiries where harm results. People will learn more useful lessons from what works than from what does not work.

Clinicians often fear an adverse outcome not so much because of the outcome, but because of the possibility of being sued, appearing in an inquiry or losing their registration. Having an awareness of the law of negligence and how this relates to duty of care can be useful. Some of these principles are outlined below.

- There can be no liability for negligence if the risk decision did not cause loss.
- If a clinician made a poor risk decision, but the harm would have happened anyway because of other factors, there is no liability in the law of negligence. (However, an inquiry, or disciplinary hearing, would still be entitled to condemn the decision-maker as the inquiry needs to consider the quality of the decision.)
- The most important requirement for the law of negligence is that the risk decision was one which no responsible body of co-professionals would have made. A judge has to decide what is professionally acceptable. The ready availability of clear, current, professionally endorsed standards and values should reduce litigation. If complainants can readily observe that the standards and practices involved in their cases were consistent with contemporary practice, they are less likely to risk being sued.[20] The benchmark was defined in *Bolam v Friern Hospital* [1957] 2 All ER 118;1 WLR 582: 'A doctor is not guilty of negligence if he has acted in accordance with a practice accepted as proper by a responsible body of medical men skilled in that particular art'.[21]

If clinicians find themselves anxious about taking risks, practice deteriorates and patients may suffer. Do risk management techniques offer any advantages? The following points outline the *benefits of risk management* and give some cause for hope.

- Risk management facilitates a pro-active approach.
- Through risk management clinicians are better prepared for crises.
- Loss of control is less likely through risk management.
- Adverse outcomes can be better prepared for.

- Risk management assists in better utilisation of resources.
- Best practice within resource limitations is possible through risk management.
- Positive outcomes from reviews and inquiries are more likely when using risk management.

Notes

1 Mullen PE 2001 Dangerousness, risk and the prediction of probability. In: *New Oxford Textbook of Psychiatry*. Oxford University Press, Oxford

2 Winestock M 1996 Risk assessment: 'a word to the wise'. *Advances in Psychiatric Treatment*, 2: 3–9.

3 Carson D 1996 Developing models of risk to aid cooperation between law and psychiatry. *Criminal Behaviour and Mental Health*, 6: 6–10.

4 Maden A 2005 Violence risk assessment: the question is not whether but how. *Psychiatric Bulletin*, 29: 121–2.

5 Maden A 2007 *Treating Violence: a Guide to Risk Management in Mental Health*. Oxford University Press, Oxford.

6 Williams J 1988 A database method for assessing and reducing human error to improve operational performance. In: Hagen W (ed) *ILEEE Fourth Conference on Human Factors and Power Plants*. Institute for Electrical and Electronic Engineers, New York: 200–31.

7 Snowden P 1997 Practical aspects of clinical risk assessment and management. *British Journal of Psychiatry*, 170 (suppl 32):32–4.

8 Matthews R 1992 Healthcare Risk Management in Dental Practice. *Healthcare Risk Management Bulletin*, 4: 7–8.

9 Snowden, above, n 7.

10 Szmukler G 2003 Blame culture, risk assessment: 'numbers' and 'values'. *Psychiatric Bulletin*, 27: 205–7

11 Royal College of Psychiatrists 2008 Rethinking Risk to Others in Mental Health Services. Final report of a scoping group. Royal College of Psychiatrists Report CR 150, June.

12 Rose D, Knight M, Fleischmann P et al 2007 Scoping Study: Public and Media Perceptions of Risk to General Public Posed by Individuals with Mental Ill Health. Service User Research Enterprise (SURE), Kings College, London.

13 Morgan JF 2007 Giving up the Culture of Blame. Briefing Document for the Royal College of Psychiatrists, February.

14 Above, n 11.

15 Adapted from: Harrison G, Risk assessment in a climate of litigation. *British Journal of Psychiatry* (Suppl), April 1997. 170: 37–9.

16 Maden, above, n 4.

17 Carson D 2008 Justifying risk decisions. *Criminal Behaviour and Mental Health (Editorial)*, 18:139–44.

18 Carson D, Bain AJ 2008 *Professional Risk and Working with People: Decision-making in Health, Social Care and Criminal Justice.* Jessica Kingsley, London.

19 Carson, above, n 17.

20 Carson, above, n 17.

21 Harrison G 1997 Risk assessment in a climate of litigation. *British Journal of Psychiatry* (Suppl), April, 170: 37–9.

2 What is risk?

It must be understood that risk cannot be eliminated entirely. To do so would be to move from risk management to certainty management, which is not possible within clinical practice.[1]

Risk is in everything that people do. Driving to work entails taking risk although often this is not consciously considered. Choosing a car or a house can be a very risky business. Buying a house requires care and assessment of all sorts of possibilities before the cheque is signed.

If there were no potential benefits to be had, people would never take any risks. For example, everyone takes risks getting to work each day and yet if they didn't take those risks, nothing would ever get done.

There will always be a degree of uncertainty about what might happen when risks are taken. For those risks that are taken every day, the likelihood of something going wrong is known to be quite low so anxiety is low. However, when it is a new risk or if the possible outcome is very severe, anxiety levels can be substantially higher.

The opposite of risk — certainty or complete safety — is something which can never be achieved in a mental health setting so clinicians will always find themselves needing to work alongside patients with a certain degree of risk and its accompanying anxiety.

For risks such as crossing the road or driving a car along the motorway, there is no need to think about how to manage the situation effectively as it has been done a thousand times before. Managing risk in a mental health setting is no different. It is primarily an exercise in decision-making. The task is to try and prevent adverse outcomes whilst maximising the likelihood of a good outcome (risks versus benefits). The process of decision-making can vary from an intuitive decision made on the run using cognitive shortcuts (heuristics;

see glossary) to a deliberate, carefully considered plan made over several days or even weeks. There are advantages and disadvantages to each process which will be explored throughout the book. With regular practice, clinicians can learn to manage risky situations effectively and minimise the risk of adverse outcomes whilst continuing to treat and care for patients.

With a clear structure to risk management, decision-making can be documented in the notes and information shared with patients and other staff. There will be less need to rely on gut feelings and intuition. Staff will be less anxious about what they are doing and will have greater potential for flexibility.

With the increasing accountability expected today, it has become more necessary to 'document our thinking for the record'.[2] Having a good structure simplifies this process substantially.

BOX 2.1 SUMMARY OF LEARNING POINTS

- If there were no potential benefits, clinicians would not need to take risks.
- Decision-making can be done quickly using cognitive short-cuts (heuristics) or be made more slowly in a deliberate and carefully weighed fashion.
- Having a clear structure to the assessment and management of risk makes practice transparent and improves communication.

Definition of risk

Dictionary definitions of risk vary, but commonly used definitions in mental health settings are:

Risk: the likelihood of an adverse event or outcome.

Risk: the possibility of incurring misfortune or loss.

Compare these definitions with the definition of chance:

Chance: the unknown and unpredictable element that causes an event to result in a certain way rather than another.

The word 'chance' is often confused with risk but it has a slightly different definition in which the outcome may be favourable.

There are three major components to any definition of risk:

1 likelihood
2 outcome: it needs to be an adverse event
3 time: how imminent is the event?

The likelihood of an event can also be considered in terms of probability, possibility, prediction and so forth.

The special quality within the definition of risk as compared to chance is that risk focuses on adverse or undesirable outcomes. It is incorrect to speak of risk when talking about an outcome which is desired. People do not talk of the risk of winning the lottery; they talk about the chance or odds of winning. Clinicians do, however, talk about the risk of a patient committing suicide and other adverse outcomes. If staff become overly occupied with suicide, homicide and self-harm it becomes easy to lose sight of the possibility of positive outcomes such as the patient getting better, or having fewer thoughts of suicide and self-harm.

When the risk may occur is not usually considered in dictionary definitions of risk. It is important, however, within mental health work to consider the time period within which risk management is being considered. The likelihood of a patient committing suicide within the next 24 hours might be very high whereas the likelihood of the same patient committing suicide within the next 2 years might be quite slim or vice versa. Whenever risk is being managed, consideration needs to be given to the imminence of the risk.

Words may come to mind when someone says 'risk', such as:

danger, threat, possibility, prospect, disaster, speculation, uncertainty, hazard, peril, gamble, jeopardy, unsafe, perilous, dodgy, touch and go, bold, daring, high gain, and so on.

Risk in mental health settings used to be synonymous with the words danger or hazard which promoted defensive practice. With increasing understanding of risk factors, the link with these words is fading and a more structured approach to the management of risk is occurring.

What are the sorts of risks?

Within mental health settings, risk is usually thought of in terms of violence, suicide or self-harm. Most people then think of risk to the patient. In practice, however, risk is a part of every decision that is made about a patient's treatment or care. If a list was drawn up of risks that existed in the workplace, it would be endless. Here are some of the risks which clinicians are involved with:

violence, death, litigation, complaints, coronial inquiries, verbal abuse, patients getting worse, burn out, sick leave, risk of relapse, insufficient resources, taking short cuts, side effects, needle stick injuries, overdose, medical complications, medication errors, social stigma, institutionalisation, stalking, intoxication, boundary problems, suicide, self-harm, and so on.

Table 2.1 Methods of categorising risk

Risks to self	Risk to others	Risk from others
• Suicide and self-harm. • Health: including alcohol and drug use, physical harm, and psychological harm. • Relapse of illness. • Quality of life: including dignity, social and financial status. • Self neglect.	• Violence: including emotional, sexual and physical violence. • Intimidation/threats. • Neglect/abuse of dependants. • Stalking/harassment. • Property damage: including arson. • Public nuisance. • Reckless behaviour: including driving.	• Harm to patients from others, especially children and elderly. • Vulnerable patients; for example, patients with mania, dementia and borderline personality disorder (BPD) are especially at risk. • Vulnerability: including exploitation, sexual abuse and violence from others. • Domestic violence.

A simple method of categorising risk is set out in Table 2.1.

Risks to whom?

Once again, the immediate thought would be risks to patients. In practice, other patients may be at risk of neglect due to more attention being paid to one particular, difficult patient or patients may be at risk of imitating self-harming behaviour displayed by another patient on the ward. In some instances, patients and clinicians may be at risk of vicarious traumatisation (see glossary) if they see an unsettling incident on a ward.

Clinicians may be at risk of burnout, stress, complaints or boundary violations.

The mental health service may be at risk of complaints, inquiries, financial costs, the effect of staff taking excessive sick leave etc. In addition, the family or community may be at risk from patients who are violent or they may be vulnerable subsequent to a patient's suicide.

What means might be used?

For violence, the history will need to include an exploration of whether the patient has a history of using weapons or whether the patient has access to weapons. For suicide, the clinical history always includes an exploration of the means that the patient has been thinking of using to complete the suicidal act.

Where might it occur?

For patients experiencing an acute episode of illness, the risk behaviours may well be more likely to occur whilst they are an inpatient in the psychiatric ward. The risks may be very much less once the patient is discharged. Some depressed patients have an increased risk of suicide at the time of discharge as they re-adapt to the home environment. For other patients, the risk may only occur in an environment where they are triggered; perhaps by seeing someone who reminds them of a previous abuser. For violence, an exploration of situations in which the patient is more likely to be violent will often yield important information.

Towards whom?

Once again this is information which will need to be considered most commonly when the risk is of violence. Often it is family members who are most at risk but for some patients experiencing persecutory delusions, it may well be members of the general public or people from certain racial groups who cannot be identified in advance. In child and adolescent mental health services, the person at risk may be the patient as a result of neglect or abuse from a parent or caregiver.

Safety

Is safety the same as risk? Safety is a word sometimes used synonymously with risk. The dictionary definition, however, is quite different:

> **Safety**: the state of being protected from or guarded against hurt or injury; freedom from danger.

In clinical practice the use of the word safety has connotations of rescuing and taking of responsibility by clinicians. From the definition, safety might be considered to be the opposite of the risk. Serious consideration should be given before the word 'safety' is used in everyday practice. Clinicians who use the word 'safety' are often anxious about their skills in risk assessment and management or are looking for a shortcut so as not to have to undertake a risk assessment. Here are two common examples of the way the word safety has been used in mental health settings.

1 'The patient couldn't guarantee their safety so I admitted them.'
   Nobody can guarantee their safety, never mind a patient with mental illness. This phrase is used less frequently nowadays but when it is used, it is unlikely that an adequate risk assessment will have been completed.

2 'The first thing I would like to consider in the management of this patient is the safety issue.'

This is a common phrase used by mental health clinicians which hopefully will become of historical interest only as the difference between risk and safety becomes more overt.

When clinicians engage in 'safety contracts' with patients, they enter into a dynamic in which an offer is made to rescue them from their torment and take responsibility. A patient who agrees to a safety contract one day may have a differing mental state the next day and no longer agree to it, but the clinician will assume the agreement is still there.[3] 'Safety contracts' were used extensively a decade ago, but fortunately have now become rare.

Eliciting guarantees of safety from the patient or developing 'no self-harm contracts' are not sufficient as sole management strategies and are not recommended.[4, 5]

BOX 2.2 WHAT IS RISK?

Learning points:
- Risk is the likelihood of an adverse outcome.
- The likelihood of risk changes over time.
- Risk is a part of every decision-making process of patient care.
- Risk involves not just the patient but the patient's family, the community, mental health staff and the mental health service.
- The use of the word 'safety' is not recommended in risk management.

Exercise

Think about the risks that you took today before you started reading this book and why you took them.

For each risk you considered, think about what might have eventuated if you hadn't taken it. Think about the benefits of taking it.

Notes

1 Royal College of Psychiatrists 2008 Rethinking Risk to Others in Mental Health Services. Final report of a scoping group. Royal College of Psychiatrists College Report CR 150, June.

2 Gutheil TG 1980 Paranoia and progress notes: a guide to forensically informed psychiatric record keeping. *Hospital and Community Psychiatry*, 31(7):479–82.

3 Bateman A, Fonagy P 2006 Mentalization Based Treatment for Borderline Personality Disorder. Oxford University Press, Oxford p 48.

4 Boyce P et al 2003 Summary of Australian and New Zealand clinical practice guidelines for the management of adult deliberate self-harm. *Australasian Psychiatry*, 11(2):150–5.

5 Rudd MD, Mandrusiak M, Joiner T 2007 The case against No-Suicide Contracts: The commitment to treatment statements as a practice alternative. *Journal of Clinical Psychology: In Session*, 62:243–51.

3 Risk factors and risk equations

To recap:

Risk = the likelihood of an adverse outcome.

It is now necessary to examine the group of two factors that, when considered together, help determine the likelihood of the event occurring.

Measuring the likelihood of the event occurring is a combination of the static risk factors and the dynamic risk factors. Or put mathematically:

Likelihood = static risk factors + dynamic risk factors

Risk factors[1]

Risk factor: Something in the patient's history or current environment or mental state which makes the adverse event more likely to occur.

Risk factors can be divided into two main categories:

1 static factors (also referred to as enduring, stable or historic factors)
2 dynamic factors (also referred to as current or variable factors).

In some forensic settings, static factors are referred to as enduring factors and dynamic factors are referred to as variable factors.

Static risk factors are factors that do not change. They are usually laid down either as a result of the patient's developmental history or are related to the patient's past external environment. Static factors give an indication of an individual's longer term *propensity for the risk*.

A comprehensive analysis of static risk factors can help ensure that clinicians take account of historical material and consider pre-existing vulnerabilities for (violence) risk when planning long-term treatment strategies.[2]

Some examples of static factors include:

- For violence: previous episodes of violence, conduct disorder and alcohol and drug history.
- For suicide: previous attempts, family history of suicide, history of mental illness.

Lists of risk factors for violence and suicide can be found in Chapter 9 (Tables 9.1 and 9.2, pp 80, 84).

The static factors set the context in which a clinician works.[3] Empirically it makes sense that the closer the patient is to these factors in time, the greater the influence they will have. However there is currently no literature available to support this. An extreme example would be of a man who was repeatedly violent in his youth but is now presenting at the age of 75. The weighting given to these factors is likely to be less than had he presented at the age of 25.

Dynamic risk factors are those factors which are more likely to change:

- as a result of alterations in the patient's mental state such as a lowering of mood (internal) and/or
- changes in the patient's external environment (situational) such as the dissolution of a relationship or loss of job.

Dynamic factors capture the fluctuating nature of risk. Dynamic factors may change in both duration and intensity. A single event may cause changes to a number of dynamic risk factors creating a change to the overall risk. Assessing the dynamic factors is essential for considering the particular conditions, patterns and circumstances that place individuals at special risk. Hanson and Harris (2000)[4] distinguished between stable and acute dynamic factors. Stable dynamic factors (e.g. traits of impulsivity or hostility) are unlikely to change over short periods of time, but can change gradually. In contrast, acute dynamic factors (e.g. drug use and mental state) can change daily or even hourly.

Further understanding of risk factors comes from knowing that certain risk factors are more likely to be relevant to certain types of risks. This knowledge is of immense importance in risk assessment as commonly occurring factors can be looked for. These factors are being refined with increasing research.

It is not sufficient to consider risk factors in isolation and manage them individually. Risk factors can affect each other in various ways. For example, one risk factor may moderate the effect of another or a second risk factor may only become relevant if the first risk factor is present. There are many possible permutations which will need to be formulated by clinicians for each patient. Whenever there are more than two causal risk factors these issues must be considered.[5] (A causal risk

BOX 3.1 THE NATURE OF RISK

Practice points
- Risk in a mental health setting is *never* static.
- The likelihood of the risk behaviour occurring is often linked to the severity of the illness.
- The nature of a patient's risk doesn't usually change; it is the likelihood and context which changes.
- The likelihood of the risk changes most with changes of the dynamic factors.
- Given the fluctuation of dynamic risk factors in patients, measures of the level of risk may have little value other than stating what it was on that particular day.
- If there is a heavy weighting of static risk factors, this is worth highlighting as the tipping point into the risk behaviour may be reached quickly.

factor is one that can be changed by manipulation and when changed can be shown to alter the risk.)

Finally, there will be risk factors that will be specific to individual patients. These have been termed 'signature risk signs' by Fluttert (2005). She states:

> In some persons with mental or personality disorder and a history of violence or self-harm, a highly specific, 'signature' set of patterns or signs may be identified (e.g. a preoccupation with certain people, or a change to a behaviour pattern), as a 'calling card' for their mental illness and the potential risk for violence to self or others.[6]

These personal signature risk signs and patterns of behaviour can be useful concepts for clinicians to consider when assessing patients. The concept of signature risk signs has been incorporated into the thinking behind 'START', an assessment tool currently being evaluated.[7] Along similar lines, the concept of 'critical risk factors' is also worth considering. These are 2–3 risk factors which will be of great importance for specific individuals and can be highlighted in management plans as flags for rapid intervention.

Looked at diagrammatically, risk factors can be presented as shown in Figure 3.1.[8]

When it comes to documenting the risk, this diagram can be referred to. The risk documentation framework used in the book is to a large degree based on this model.

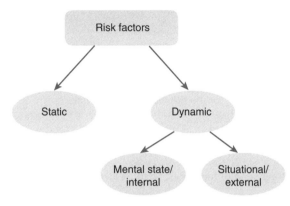

Figure 3.1 Diagramatic representation of risk factors

BOX 3.2 CLINICAL TIP

- When assessing risk, look for patterns of risk factors which repeat themselves in the history. When the same risk factors occur repeatedly, the same risk behaviour is more likely to occur.
- Look for 'signature risk signs' that are specific to the patient.

Example 1 — violence risk factors

Jimmy was brought up in a violent household (static factor). He was diagnosed with conduct disorder when 11 (static factor). He is currently experiencing command auditory hallucinations (dynamic factor — mental state) and wants to kill the Prime Minister. He lives down the road from Parliament (dynamic factor — situational) and has stopped his medication (dynamic factor — situational).

When knowledge of the static risk factors is combined with that of the dynamic risk factors, an estimation of the likelihood of the risk occurring can be made. This can be used to help plan an intervention in the here and now. Efforts can then be made to reduce the likelihood of dynamic risk factors occurring again or if they do, early interventions can be implemented.

The synthesis of the static and dynamic risk factors combines to give the current 'risk state'.[9, 10] The risk state is a term used in some literature to describe the likelihood of the risk occurring at a given time.

> **BOX 3.3 RISK FACTORS**
>
> - Static factors are static and stable and do not usually change. They indicate the individual's propensity for the risk.
> - Dynamic factors can be related to either the mental state (internal) or the external environment (situational). Dynamic factors account for the fluctuating level of risk.

The graphs in Figures 3.2 and 3.3 help describe the idea of risk being a synthesis of static and dynamic factors. The second graph also shows how the likelihood of the risk occurring can change quickly.

Example 2[11]

Figure 3.2 shows graphically a patient with chronic depression. The patient is a 54-year-old woman who has had recurring episodes of major depression throughout her adult life. Treatment has included antidepressants, supportive psychotherapy and electroconvulsive therapy (ECT). On three occasions she has attempted to kill herself. On the last occasion she was found accidentally by a hunter as she was gassing herself in

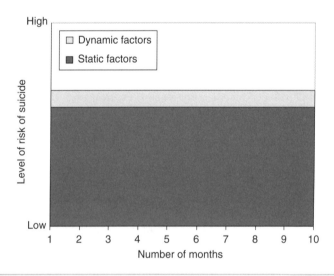

Figure 3.2 Chronic high risk due to static risk factors

her car, which was parked deep in the woods. She has a lot of static risk factors: three previous suicide attempts, physical illness, sexual abuse as a child, family history of mental disorder and her own history of mental illness. These leave her especially vulnerable to the risk of relapse and further suicidality if there is a small change in her dynamic factors. This needs to be considered when assessing and managing the risk.

Precipitating events can 'tip the balance'[12] easily into a risk event and may only need to be minor in this example. It may be necessary to review the patient frequently as it will only take a small change in the dynamic factors for the pathway into suicide to be completed. Being mindful of the weighting given to each of the static and dynamic factors is going to be important in the assessment of what it takes for a patient's suicidal intent to be realised. For individual patients, there are likely to be specific releasing factors (signature risk signs) clustered into two or three critical risk factors that tip the patient over into the risk behaviour.

Example 3

Figure 3.3 shows a very different scenario. This patient is a young man of 25 who is 'happily married'. He has no previous history of mental illness but does drink in a binge pattern. Over the course of 10 days, he loses his job on day 1, his father has a heart attack on day 5 and his wife confesses she has been having an affair with his brother on day 8! This

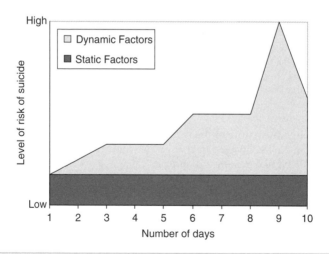

Figure 3.3 Rapid onset and partial resolution of dynamic risk factors

patient has very few static factors for suicide which would usually pose little risk but over the period of a few days, he has a series of life events which destabilise his mental state and raise the risk of suicide substantially. He has dynamic risk factors of loss, recent adverse events, rage and feeling abandoned. On day 9 the risk peaks and by day 10 there has been some resolution of the dynamic factors and the risk rapidly reduces. In Chapter 9 there is a list of risk factors for suicide (Table 9.1, p 80) which will help when doing assessments.

In this example, the path towards a possible suicide attempt is clear and rapid: close levels of observation and support will be required. In the longer term, however, once the acute episode has settled, it is unlikely that the patient will need the frequency of review which was necessary in example 2.

One of the difficulties in assessing risk within a mental health context is that the likelihood of the event happening (the risk state) is *never* static. The likelihood will vary with any change in the risk factors.

Thus the word 'likelihood' in the equation

Risk = the *likelihood* of an adverse outcome.

is *NOT* a constant at all but can change daily and even hourly. The likelihood of the risk behaviour occurring will fluctuate with time, context and intervention.

EXAMPLE OF THE LIKELIHOOD (RISK STATE) CHANGING

Andrew is usually a mild mannered, placid person who wouldn't harm a fly. He decides to try some methamphetamine (speed) and within an hour is feeling very violent and aggressive. Four hours later the likelihood of violence lessens as the drug wears off.

Although the nature of the risk (e.g. in this case violence) is unlikely to change, the likelihood can change enormously. When assessing risk, it is a little bit like making a diagnosis: a diagnosis is only a snapshot in time. A risk assessment is similarly a snapshot in time and its predictive quality weakens with every passing hour and day. A risk assessment will give the indicators and patterns of what makes the risk behaviour more likely to occur. Risk management involves an assessment of the current circumstances whenever the patient is seen. This includes a review of the patient's mental state and the patient's external environment; that is, no different to routine and usual clinical practice.

Level of risk

Level of risk = likelihood × severity of consequences

Sometimes clinicians have to work in environments or situations when the levels of risk are described as being high. It is useful not to forget that there can be rewards even when the risks are high; for example, 'She risked her life to save a friend'. Good treatment may involve living with high levels of risk.

To understand levels of risk, consider an outcome with a very, very low likelihood such as a meteor falling onto earth. This could have very severe consequences (the death of millions). If one was to add the likelihood which is very low and the consequences which are very high, the level would immediately be seen as extreme but when the two factors are multiplied, the event would still be seen as being a low to moderate risk rather than an extreme risk. This is important to understand in mental health work. Many of the risks which occur in this field have substantial consequences but the likelihood of them occurring is often quite low. The 'base rates' (the frequency in which an event occurs in a given population) of suicide and violence are both low in the general population and even within the population of mental health patients they are still quite low.

Table 3.1 demonstrates the changeability of the level of risk with fluctuations of likelihood and consequences.

Table 3.1 Changes in level of risk

Likelihood	Consequences				
	Insignificant	Minor	Moderate	Major	Catastrophic
A (almost certain)	H	H	E	E	E
B (likely)	M	H	H	E	E
C (moderate)	L	M	H	E	E
D (unlikely)	L	L	M	H	E
E (rare)	L	L	M	H	H

Legend:
E: Extreme risk
H: High risk
M: Moderate risk
L: Low risk

An example from clinical practice is nausea which is a common side effect of the drug naltrexone. The likelihood may be moderate but the consequences are minor so the level of risk is felt to be low.

It is useful at this stage to consider the various components of the level of risk which will lead to a clinician trying to determine whether it is high, moderate or low.

How imminent is the risk?

The number of static risk factors that the patient has will only have a small effect on the imminence of the risk. The static risk factors relate more to the propensity for the risk behaviour. A rule of thumb is that the more static factors a patient has, the lower the threshold will be for the risk behaviour to occur. However, this is invariably trumped by the dynamic risk factors which in the here and now are of much more relevance.

For example, when a student believes that people are plotting against him, feels threatened and develops a delusional belief that the world will end if he does not kill his teacher, the imminence is much greater than when the patient's psychosis has been adequately treated. The other component to this dilemma of imminence is the environment which the patient is in. Imminence is often greater within acute psychiatric units than the community as a result of both the environment of inpatient units and the degree of illness. However, in the example of the student, the imminence may be greater in the classroom or the teacher's home.

Each time a patient is seen, an assessment will be made of the imminence of the risk occurring. On an inpatient unit this may occur every 5 minutes. In an outpatient setting, the judgment may only occur every 6 months. The greater the number of risk factors, especially *critical risk factors*, which are present at any given time, the greater the likelihood that the risk is imminent.

What are the consequences?

If the consequence is considered minor — for example, a mild headache for a few hours when taking a new medication — but the likelihood is high, there is little cause for concern. If the consequence is a suicide but the likelihood is moderate, everyone worries more.

High, moderate or low risk?

To recap: when a risk is designated as having a certain level — high, moderate or low — this is a product of the likelihood of it occurring and the consequences of it occurring.

BOX 3.4 CLINICAL TIP

A common cause for the level of risk changing acutely is anything which can change levels of consciousness. This can include:
- delirium
- evening time for patients with dementia
- disinhibiting effects of substances, especially alcohol.

Assessments of the level of risk are frequently made in forensic settings when predictions are made for the future. They can also be used in everyday practice to indicate the level in the here and now. Once an assessment is completed, the documentation of the level of the risk can become a big problem. For example, if a patient is described as being a high risk, that may be true one day but not the next. The changeability of dynamic factors is of greatest relevance here. (Obviously, if Andrew from the example on page 24 takes methamphetamine again, the aggressive feelings are likely to return and the level of risk will be higher for a few hours.) Alternatively, a patient with a lot of static risk factors may be a high risk of displaying the risk behaviour at some time in the future and may need closer monitoring. When levels of risk are used in routine documentation, this should automatically generate a degree of monitoring with specified review dates built in to ensure that the level is reviewed. This is routine practice in acute psychiatric units and for a lot of forensic patients. If levels of risk are not clearly defined and standardised, neither the clinicians nor their family will be able to give any meaning to them. One person's definition will differ from another's which will lead to confusion.

Using levels of risk may cause problems, however. If a patient is described as being high risk, the label tends to stick and may cause stigma to the patient and prejudice for clinicians; never mind the problems that may arise later when efforts are made to explain management decisions if there is a bad outcome. If a patient is termed high risk, the risk thereafter is of staff being held responsible if the patient converts their risk factors into action. This tends to lead to defensive practice which is not without its own risk. It is important for clinicians to remember to involve the patient and their family in the management of the risk. By designating the risk as being high, there is a tendency for clinicians to take the responsibility away from the patient. This must be guarded against.

Describing a patient as high risk may not be conducive to developing a therapeutic alliance as there will be a tendency to be rejecting of patients. Compliance with treatment will be less likely. The stigma attached to patients if they are categorised as being high risk should be avoided where possible. Another argument to be made against using a focus on level of risk is that resources may be diverted towards those deemed to be at highest risk and away from those with other mental illnesses.[13]

Risk assessment and management plans should be explicit about the time period for which they are made. To set a valid schedule for assessing and monitoring risk state, a clinician must have a sense for the speed at which an individual's most important dynamic factors will change.[14]

Documenting a patient as being 'high, moderate or low risk' is an absolute measurement. Using a risk management plan which makes an argument for a certain degree of monitoring when certain conditions are met is more qualitative and relative. Given the ever-changing likelihood of the event occurring, this approach may well be considered to be more useful to general mental health clinicians than absolute statements of level of risk.

BOX 3.5 PRACTICE TIP

High risk usually refers to the imminence of the risk behaviour occurring or to the seriousness and/or consequences of the behaviour occurring. Often the documentation of the level of risk is limited to a tick box which provides no useful information to anybody and simply puts the clinician at risk.

A simple and effective way of documenting the level of risk for the future is to utilise a narrative form of documentation to qualify terms such as 'high' and 'low' along the lines of:

The patient will pose a higher risk when he is acutely psychotic and perceives himself to be threatened by others. At these times his impulsivity is greatly increased and he will have a low threshold for violence, especially as he has utilised violence repeatedly in the past.

The essence of these two sentences is a description of the patient's individual dynamic risk factors taking past patterns into account. This can be used for future assessments and in generating treatment for his psychosis.

Using standardised tools such as the Historical/Clinical/Risk Management 20-item (HCR 20)[15] help identify the level of risk but will not necessarily add anything to the meaning of the risk behaviour for the patient, which will be specific to them.

Finally, clinicians, their managers and health trusts run the risk of using levels of risk to become agents of social control.

> If the interests of the patient are given primacy, there is little problem. However, violence risk assessment processes may be utilised with public protection as the primary goal. This is ethically troubling territory for the mental health professional, even more so where the processes rely entirely on static risk factors that are not open to therapeutic change.[16]

It is sometimes too easy to say that the patient is high risk and needs to be detained involuntarily without pursuing other options. This is sometimes used as an anxiety reduction tool for clinicians (secondary risk management). The obverse side of this coin is to treat the patient in the least restrictive setting and ignore the risk. Good risk management practice will minimise the likelihood of either of these polarities being taken unwittingly. Remember:

- 'primary risk management' is the term for managing risk as it pertains to the patient
- 'secondary risk management' is the term used to describe risk management undertaken to reduce clinician anxiety but not reduce the risk for the patient.[17]

Summary

- Levels of risk can be useful in setting up systems for regular monitoring of patients.
- Levels of risk need to be clearly defined for each risk group and possibly for different settings in order to be meaningful.
- Levels of risk can identify patients from whom the public needs to be protected. (Some people suggest that this is using risk management to be an agent of social control.)
- Using levels of risk can help identify patients who need greater numbers of resources. The risk here is that other patients miss out.
- Documentation of level of risk may cause stigma to the patient.

Exercise — level of risk changing over time

Richard is a 42-year-old man with a severe depressive illness. He presents to the crisis team clutching a knife and tells you that his family would be better off without him.

1 What is the likelihood of Richard committing suicide tonight?

Two days later, Richard is an inpatient in the psychiatric unit. He is beginning to question whether his family would be better off without him.

2 Has the likelihood of risk changed?

Three weeks later, Richard is less depressed. You have had a meeting with Richard's family and discussed his prognosis and the likelihood of him having a relapse of his depressive illness in the future and the possibility of him committing suicide at some stage in the future.

3 Has the likelihood of risk changed?

4 Has the nature of the risk changed?

Refer to Appendix 3 for possible answers.

BOX 3.6 PRACTICE TIPS

- A narrative approach indicating in which situations a patient may be at higher or lower risk is useful. It allows for identification of times of increased risk and for interventions to be planned.
- If the risk is documented as high, moderate or low, frequency and levels of monitoring need to be specified and review dates included. To set a valid schedule for assessing and monitoring risk state, a clinician must have a sense for the speed at which an individual's most important dynamic factors will change.
- The decision whether to document level of risk may be made for you by your managers. If not, think carefully about the clinical usefulness of documenting a level of risk at this time and whether it will help your patient. It is always useful to ask the question 'Is the risk being rated as high for the benefit of the patient or the protection of the public?'

Note: It should not be forgotten that to ignore the seriousness of the potential for the risk behaviour is also poor practice and must be avoided. It should not be forgotten that clinicians also do patients a disservice if they are allowed to pose a threat to the public.

BOX 3.7 SUMMARY OF RISK EQUATIONS

- Risk = the likelihood of an adverse outcome.
- Likelihood = static risk factors + dynamic risk factors.
- Level of risk = likelihood × severity of consequences.

Notes

1 Bouch J, Marshall JJ 2005 Suicide Risk: structured professional judgment. *Advances in Psychiatric Treatment*, 11:84–91.

2 Mullen P 2000 Dangerousness, risk and the prediction of probability. In: Gelder M, Lopez-Ibor JJ, Andreasen NC (eds) *New Oxford Textbook of Psychiatry*, Oxford University Press, Oxford, pp 2066–78.

3 Maden A 2007 Treating Violence: a guide to risk management in mental health. Oxford University Press, Oxford.

4 Hanson RK, Harris AJR 2000 Where should we intervene? Dynamic predictors of sexual offense recidivism. *Criminal Justice and Behavior*, 27:6–35.

5 Kraemer HC 2003 Current concepts of risk in psychiatric disorders. *Current Opinion in Psychiatry*, 16(4):421–30.

6 Fluttert F 2005 Nursing study of personal based 'early recognition and early intervention' schemes in forensic care. Paper presented at 5th Annual Conference, International Association of Forensic Mental Health Services, Melbourne, April.

7 Webster CD, Nicholls TL, Martin ML, Desmarais SL, Brink J 2006 Short-Term Assessment of Risk and Treatability (START): The case for a New Structured Professional Judgment Scheme. *Behavioural Science and the Law*, 24:747–66.

8 Adapted from: New Zealand Ministry of Health 2006 Assessment and Management of Risk to Others Guidelines; Development of Training Toolkit; and Trainee Workbook. New Zealand Ministry of Health. Online. Available: www.mhwd.govt.nz (accessed 12 Oct 2009).

9 Skeem JL, Mulvey E 2002 Monitoring the violence potential of mentally disordered offenders being treated in the community. In: Buchanan A (ed.) *Care of the Mentally Disordered Offender in the Community*, Oxford Press, New York, pp 111–42.

10 Douglas KS, Skeem JL 2005 Violence risk assessment. Getting specific about being dynamic. *Psychology, Public Policy and Law*, 11(3):347–83.

11 Adapted from Bouch J, Marshall JJ 2005 Suicide risk: structured professional judgment. *Advances in Psychiatric Treatment*, 11:84–91.

12 New Zealand Ministry of Health 1998 Guidelines for Clinical Risk Assessment and Management in Mental Health Services. New Zealand Ministry of Health, p 17.

13 Szmukler G 2003 Risk Assessment: 'numbers' and values. *Psychiatric Bulletin*, 27:205–7.

14 Douglas & Skeem, above, n 10.

15 Webster CD, Douglas KF, Eaves D et al 1997 *HCR-20: Assessing Risk of Violence* (version 2). Mental Health Law and Policy Institute, Simon Fraser University, Vancouver.

16 Carroll A 2007 Are violence risk assessment tools clinically useful? *Australian and New Zealand Journal of Psychiatry*, 41:301–7.

17 Undrill G 2007 The risks of risk assessment. *Advances in Psychiatric Treatment*, 13:291–7.

4 Understanding the risk

It is not sufficient to simply identify the risk and risk factors associated in order to manage the risk. It is also necessary to identify patterns which make the risk behaviour more likely and, to do this, the previous episodes of risk behaviour will need to be explored in as much detail as possible. It is from the analysis of previous episodes of risk behaviour that the patterns will begin to emerge. Further information which will yield more information about the patterns of risk are the elements of personal meaning which a patient will attach to the risk.

From the identification of patterns and understanding of the meaning attached to the risk, *critical risk factors* may be identified.

The process for exploring this information is termed the 'anamnestic analysis' (anamnesis — the recalling of things past). The term anamnesis has a long history in mental health work and refers more specifically to a reconstruction of the historical development of the behaviour.[1] A structure for this aspect of the risk assessment, such as a chain analysis[2] or functional analysis,[3] may be used. The behaviour is examined step-by-step as closely as possible to try and pick up the antecedents as well as the behavioural and emotional consequences to the behaviour.

There are three main ways in which this information can be found:

1 taking the history from the patient
2 discussion with relatives and friends, other health care providers and so forth
3 examination of previous case files, criminal records and so forth.

It is very common for some of this information to be gleaned from previous case files. Taking the collateral history is a routine part of history taking within mental health practice and this is no different when undertaking a risk assessment.

Exploring past episodes of risk behaviour and identifying patterns

If the risk behaviour has occurred before, it is extremely likely that there is a pattern to the behaviour. Either the external events are being repeated (e.g. loss of job, loss of relationship) or the patient's mental state is the same (e.g. relapse of psychosis with command hallucinations). Sometimes the external events will cause a relapse of the patient's illness or a relapse will create a change in the external environment making the risk behaviour more likely to occur.

Within the risk assessment, looking for patterns to the risk behaviour is a very important guide for future risk management.

The patterns usually relate to the dynamic factors. The discovery of these patterns is important for two reasons:

1 if the external environment and/or mental state match previous patterns, the level of risk is likely to be high
2 the patterns identified will lay the foundation for future interventions. From here, triggers and early warning signs can be identified, which can ultimately lead to relapse prevention work.

The importance of exploring previous risk episodes in detail cannot be emphasised enough.

The history of past episodes of risk behaviours needs to include:

- the mental state at the time — whether it occurred in the context of illness
- treatment at the time — whether medication was being taken
- the social circumstances at the time — when, where and to whom it happened
- whether substance use was involved.

Example 1

If Bobby discontinues his medication, stops washing himself and becomes pre-occupied with the Old Testament in the Bible, it is likely that his delusional pre-occupation with Satan has returned. This has been linked to his violent outbursts in the past.

Comment: although the major risk factor leading to violence is a delusional pre-occupation with Satan, this may not be evident to his clinicians as Bobby may not speak about it. The risk factors of stopping medication, not washing and reading the Old Testament together is the pattern which is of more use.

Example 2 Suicidal intent in the context of intoxication

It is not unusual to come across patients who only express suicidal intent in the context of intoxication.

Emma is a 28-year-old woman who has a binge pattern of alcohol abuse. She has co-morbid problems of dysthymia and she also has post-traumatic stress disorder (PTSD). From time to time, her intrusive memories of her trauma (a rape at the age of 18) become more pervasive and to manage these memories, she often turns to alcohol. She describes her depression as getting the better of her at these times and she is clear that she is only ever actively suicidal when drunk. She has now made three substantive efforts to kill herself when intoxicated. When each suicide attempt was explored in detail with Emma, several recurring themes/patterns emerged: intoxication, intrusive memories and difficulties within her relationship with her boyfriend. These were explored further when her boyfriend's perspective was heard (with Emma present) and when her previous notes were reviewed.

Emma was able to identify these patterns at an earlier stage as time went by and was able to request support before she slipped into an alcohol binge.

This exploration will yield the most important patterns of risk factors particular to that patient — the signature risk signs and/or the critical risk factors and may highlight the pathway that leads to the risk behaviour. 'Risk scenarios' — situations or states of mind when the risk is more likely to occur — are another way in which the patterns leading to the risk behaviour are sometimes described.

BOX 4.1 ANAMNESTIC ANALYSIS OF RISK

Practice points
- A detailed analysis of past episodes of the risk behaviour should always be undertaken.
- *Patterns* of risk behaviours should be identified; *critical risk factors* and/or *signature risk signs* for individual patients can be identified from the patterns.
- A chain or functional analysis of events, thoughts and emotions leading up to the risk behaviour and following on from it can help in understanding the function of the behaviour.
- The exploration of the function can assist in elucidating pathways and patterns for the risk behaviour.

Not infrequently, there will be substantial resistance to an exploration of the history of the risk behaviour. A good example would be the patient who has committed sexual crimes. For a patient to discuss this with a clinician is extremely difficult and the process may take not just weeks but often months. Nonetheless, the same process should occur and as more meaning is obtained by both the patient and the clinician, a better understanding can be had of the drivers of the risk behaviour.

The function of risk behaviours — more detailed analysis

A further component of the assessment of risk is the exploration of the function of the risk. This can also be considered as an exploration of the meaning of, motivation behind, or purpose of the risk behaviour.

An example is of a patient who has a delusional belief that if he doesn't kill his mother, the world will end. For this poor man, the function of acting on the delusional belief would be to save the world even if it means sacrificing his mother, and for him, the risk behaviour has substantial meaning.

The risk behaviour now becomes understandable. It puts the behaviour firmly back into the context of the patient's illness and allows for an exploration of treatment modalities as well as ways of limiting the opportunities for the patient to act on the impulse. Making sense of the risk behaviour with the patient is a good way of improving rapport.

Another example is the patient with borderline personality disorder (BPD) who cuts herself in order to be able to feel emotion. Knowing that she does not have any other skills for the expression of emotion makes the behaviour understandable even if there is a risk of exsanguination from deep cuts. (This example becomes complicated as there is often an associated desire for death or peace at the time of the cutting which adds further meaning to the risk behaviour.)

A further example would be a patient who is violent but only in certain circumscribed situations. Exploring this and discovering that his father had sadistic tendencies, which the patient is repeating, provides a meaning and understanding to the violent behaviour which can be utilised in treatment.

Exploring the function of the risk behaviour can be broken down into two parts. The first part is looking into the patient's thoughts and feelings before the risk behaviour occurs. In the first example, the risk factor of the delusional belief is already present but for the patient to act on the delusional belief, he will need to go through the anguish of trying to work out whether he should kill his mother or not. In the example of the patient who is only violent in certain situations, a similar exercise would be undertaken of exploring the thoughts and feelings which are occurring for the patient prior to the risk behaviour occurring.

The second part is looking at the patient's thoughts and feelings after the risk behaviour has happened. This is more relevant for those risks where the behaviour is reinforcing in some way for the patient. For those patients where the risk behaviour is reinforcing, there may be immense difficulty in attempting to reduce the risk as there will be barriers erected to prevent this from happening. As well as documenting the meaning or purpose of the risk behaviour, it is important to explore whether there are any reinforcers of it.

For example, a patient says that he is more likely to assault his girlfriend if he is not given benzodiazepines. The threats of assault are regarded as the risk but there will be resistance to the management of them by the patient because this would cause his supply of benzodiazepines to dry up. The real problem is the patient's dependence on benzodiazepines. As treatment proceeds, there is a possibility that the threats will increase before they are extinguished.

Another common example is when a patient with BPD finds their self-harming behaviour reinforcing as it reduces their distress, causes their family to be worried about them and for mental health professionals to display rescuing behaviour by admitting them to hospital.

In both of these examples, there will be substantial conscious and unconscious resistance to having the risk behaviour reduced. This resistance can also be seen in clinicians who will need to sit with higher levels of risk and anxiety in the short term in order for the problem behaviours to be successfully managed.

To further complicate matters, sometimes there is substantial ambivalence. In the latter example, a part of the patient may want to 'die' (often there is a desire for death, peace and a break from the torment) whilst another part will want the rescuing behaviour of family and mental health staff.

Patients with an alcohol or drug disorder or with a coexisting mental illness and substance abuse create further complications. Sometimes distress will be alleviated by using substances which then become reinforcing. The difficulty is that substance use can become risky behaviour in its own right.

This is explored further in Chapter 16, Psychodynamic principles and boundary issues.

BOX 4.2 CLINICAL TIP

Risk behaviours in mental health settings are invariably associated with fear. It is unusual for patients not to experience fear as a result of their altered mental state. This is certainly the case for patients who are suicidal or who are preoccupied with self-harm thoughts but it is also very common in patients who demonstrate violence. It would not be unusual for a patient to display violence as the only way that they feel they can protect themselves from a perceived threat. Exploring a patient's fear will help in understanding the function of the risk behaviour.

For the patient to be able to understand the function of the risk is often the beginning of a therapeutic shift for the patient and their family. As a component of risk assessment and management, this cannot be undertaken without the patient (and their family when appropriate) being an active participant. This discussion during the assessment often becomes the starting point for the development of interventions and a shared perspective of the risk. In conjunction with the management of the risk factors, clinicians can then plan interventions with the patient based on the knowledge gained and the risk is reduced.

BOX 4.3 PATTERNS OF RISK BEHAVIOUR

Practice points
The following four points need to be covered when looking for the patterns of risk:
1 the mental state at the time — whether it occurred in the context of illness
2 treatment at the time — whether medication was being taken
3 the social circumstances at the time — what was happening, and when, where and to whom it happened
4 whether substance use was involved.

Notes
1 Jung CG 1934 *Collected Works. The Development of Personality* (vol 17), pp 177–80.

2 Linehan MM 1993 *Cognitive Behavioural Treatment of Borderline Personality Disorder.* The Guilford Press, New York.

3 Sturmey P 1996 *Functional Analysis in Clinical Psychology.* Wiley, New York.

5 The context of risk

Knowledge and clinical skill are helpful but do not inoculate the clinician against the discomfort of uncertainty.[1]

The most important context in which the assessment and management of risk occurs is within the relationship between the clinician and the patient. Other relationships of importance are the relationship between the clinician and the wider family and the relationships that the clinician has with the rest of his/her team. Best practice in the assessment and management of risk is to include the patient and the family at all stages wherever possible. Where all parties have a shared understanding of the risk, the risk factors and the proposed interventions, the best outcomes can be expected.

As well as the quality of the relationship with the patient and their family, the clinician needs to firmly consider the risk within the context of the patient's illness. If clinicians focus completely on the risk, they may lose sight of the disease process and if they focus completely on the disease process, they may become blasé about the risk. Managing both concurrently becomes the task.

If risk management is taken out of the context of clinical management, it will lose its meaning and promote defensive practice and the risk of making the patient worse occurs.

Remember:

Clinical risk assessment should be motivated primarily by the intention to provide a patient with better treatment and care.

These two positions can be shown diagrammatically, as seen in Figure 5.1.

Other contextual factors are not necessarily related to the patient or the relationship that the clinician has with the patient. There may be personal factors with the

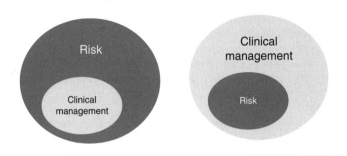

Figure 5.1 Risk versus clinical management as the main focus

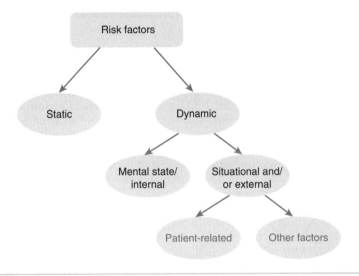

Figure 5.2 Flow chart — further differentiation of risk factors

clinician, dynamic problems within the clinician's team and difficulties accessing resources in which to manage the risk.

It is necessary to expand the previous thinking about the dynamic situational factors and divide these into patient-related factors and non-patient related factors (see the flow chart in Figure 5.2).

In the 'other factors' circle, consideration can be given to other issues that may influence the risk and the outcome. These may include:

- situational factors that are not directly related to the patient but are more related to the wider social environment, such as culture, ethnicity, religion, psycho-social influences, and so forth
- physical environment concerns; for example, the layout of an inpatient ward, whether a potentially violent patient is being seen in a forensic setting or in their home, and so forth
- protective factors
- personal (clinician) responses to the risk (see Chapter 6)
- multidisciplinary team (MDT) and other systemic responses to the risk (see Chapter 7)
- resources available for managing the risk and the clinical condition.

Cultural, ethnic and psycho-social factors affecting risk

These factors can have a substantial influence on the likelihood of an adverse outcome. Culture has many different meanings and can vary from a small cultural group such as a gang to a worldwide religion. It is important for clinicians to be aware of cultural factors which may be of relevance in their locality. This is especially the case in larger cities where refugees are more likely to live. Becoming aware of different religious belief structures and special factors relating to indigenous populations is also of relevance. It is usually possible to utilise interpreters, religious and indigenous leaders and so forth to help in these situations.

These factors can be considered from different perspectives: religion, ethnicity, cultural stigma and refugees.

- **Religion**. Religion has long been linked to causation of violence, to war and to suicide. Over thousands of years, wars have been fought in the name of religion and this continues today. Terror sects fight in the name of religion and some religions have fanatical offshoots in which violence is sanctioned. Other religious groups in the last five decades have been associated with mass suicide; for example, the Jonestown mass suicide in 1978.[3]

  Religion can also be linked to protective factors. Catholicism classically was perceived as being a protective factor for suicide. It is generally recognised that a strong faith does protect one from suicide to a certain extent.[4]

- **Ethnicity and psycho-social influences**. Certain ethnic groups in different countries have a higher risk of completed suicide. Dependent on country, different ethnic groups may be more vulnerable.[5] There are also some ethnic groups in which alcohol use is problematical and this can be linked to increased risk of suicide.[6] It pays to take note of regional ethnic variations related to risk. Some indigenous populations are at higher risk of suicide. In 1995, a Royal Commission Report estimated that suicide rates across all age groups of Aboriginal people were on average about three times higher than in the non-Aboriginal population.[7] Recently, a high female suicide rate in China has been noted and is considered to be related to particular pressures on women in modern Chinese society.[8]

A particular example of violence linked to ethnicity is the rate of female feticide (the death of a fetus) and infanticide in India as a result of the preference for boy children.[9]

- **Cultural stigma**. In some cultures, there may be cultural distrust and stigma associated with health-seeking behaviour.[10] This may occur especially in Third World countries when Western practices are introduced.
- **Refugees**. This group can also be very vulnerable. High rates of post-traumatic stress disorder (PTSD) in refugees[11] and difficulty integrating with different cultural mores can raise risk.

Particular forms of risk behaviour can also be culturally determined. For example, self-immolation (burning of oneself) in India is heavily weighted towards women in the age group 15–34.[12] This is not necessarily related to any religious belief but possibly a function of societal belief structures. It is also necessary to consider local cultural variations which may have a bearing on risk. For example, it is not unusual for gangs to congregate in certain cities and towns. Considering gang affiliation and whether there is a subculture of sanctioned violence will be of relevance.

The physical environment of risk

The physical environment in which the patient is being treated will influence the likelihood of the risk behaviour occurring. The likelihood of a patient being violent in an inpatient unit may be much higher than if they were living in the family home or vice versa. However, the consequences of violence in the family home, if it occurs, may be much more severe. The layout of psychiatric units also has a bearing on the likelihood of risk behaviours occurring. Units with open spaces and with good facilities for observation are likely to have fewer episodes of violence.

When a patient in whom there is a risk of violence is interviewed, is this undertaken by a clinician on their own sitting nearest the door?

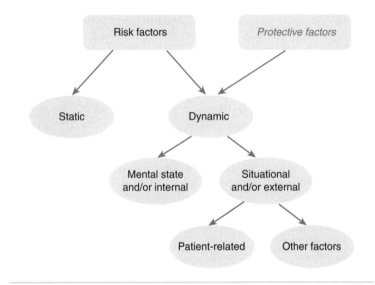

Figure 5.3 Flow chart — the influence of protective factors on risk

For a suicidal patient, does the physical layout of the ward enable unobtrusive observation to occur? In virtually every clinical situation, the physical environment will be of some importance.

This topic will be covered in more detail in Chapter 12, Risk management.

Protective factors

Adding in an assessment of the protective factors is a central component of risk assessment which is sometimes forgotten. Protective factors are usually linked to dynamic risk factors such as compliance with medication and family support. Exploring protective factors with the patient and their family allows for development of rapport when discussing the difficult topic of risk, provides hope and can also move the focus away from the risk behaviour if the interview is getting difficult. When talking about protective factors, the discussion can also usefully include an exploration of early warning signs and triggers.

The flow chart from Figure 5.2 can be expanded again (see Figure 5.3).

Notes

1 Miller MC, Tabakin R, Schimmel J 2000 Managing risk when risk is greatest. *Harvard Rev Psychiatry*, 8:154–9.

2 Mullen PE 2001 Dangerousness, risk and the prediction of probability. *New Oxford Textbook of Psychiatry*. Oxford University Press, Oxford.

3 Reiterman T, Jacobs J 1982 *Raven: The Untold Story of Rev. Jim Jones and His People*. EP Dutton Publishers, Boston.

4 Goldney RD 2008 *Suicide Prevention*. Oxford University Press, Oxford.

5 Bhui KS, McKenzie K 2008 Rates and risk factors by ethnic group for suicides within a year of contact with mental health services in England and Wales. *Psychiatric Services*, 59(4):414–20.

6 Centres for Disease Control and Prevention (CDC) 2009 Alcohol and suicide among racial/ethnic populations in 17 States, 2005–2006. *MMWR — Morbidity and Mortality Weekly Report*, 58(23):637–41.

7 Suicide among Aboriginal People: Royal Commission Report. Prepared by Nancy Miller Chenier. Political and Social Affairs Division, 23 February 1995.

8 Goldney, above, n 4.

9 Sumner M 2009 The unknown genocide: how one country's culture is destroying the girl child. *International Journal of Nursing Practice*, 15(2):65–8.

10 Goldston DB, Molock SD, Whitbeck LB, Leslie B, Murakami JL, Zayas LH, Gordon CN 2008 Cultural considerations in adolescent suicide prevention and psychosocial treatment. *American Psychologist*, 63(1):14–31.

11 Corales TA 2005 *Trends in Post-Traumatic Stress Disorder Research*. Nova Science Publishers, Hauppauge, New York.

12 Sanghavi P, Bhalla K, Das V 2009 Fire-related deaths in India in 2001: a retrospective analysis of data. *The Lancet*, 373(9671):1282–8.

6 Personal (clinician) responses to risk

Within health care, clinicians are exposed to risks every day. Patients are exposed to risk, clinicians take risks and they sometimes put themselves at risk. Occasionally (perhaps often) clinicians feel that they carry all the risk or they find themselves saying, 'We can't take the risk'. Murphy (2002) comments, 'Apart from the need to assess and manage risk, it also has an emotional component for all concerned and often a judgmental aspect.'[1] Undrill (2007) says, 'Risk assessment has become a large and anxiety provoking part of the work of many psychiatrists.'[2]

Personal response to risk may vary from moment-to-moment and day-to-day. Sometimes it is easy to manage the risk and at other times clinicians may be more likely to avoid dealing with problems. In other situations, clinicians may be surrounded by so much risk that they become blasé about it.

The risk thermostat[3]

The risk thermostat is a conceptual, qualitative model of how behaviour in risky situations is influenced by perceptions and attitudes. Cultural theory explains risk-taking behaviour by the operation of filters. It postulates that behaviour is governed by the probable costs and benefits of alternative courses of action which are perceived through filters formed from all the previous incidents and associations in the risk-taker's life. This is shown diagrammatically in Figure 6.1.

Exercise 1

Below is a continuum which can be useful to consider when faced with a risk problem. The continuum characterises the alternative courses of action which will have been considered when risk decisions were taken previously. It allows for a consideration of where your risk thermostat is set at any given time and how the setting may change in different circumstances.

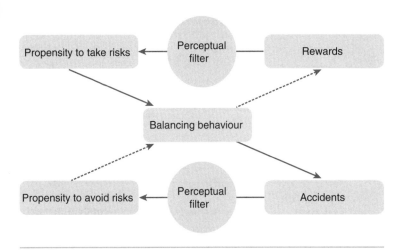

Figure 6.1 **The risk thermostat**

Imagine a recent episode in which you managed risk and ask yourself where you were on this continuum. Was the issue being managed by being risk-avoidant or risk-taking or was it being managed in a balanced way which required you or your team to be in the middle of the continuum?

Propensity to	Propensity to
avoid risks	take risks

Figure 6.2 **Risk continuum**

Most clinicians move up and down this continuum depending on many different factors. On the whole, it is easier to be risk-avoidant or blithely risk-taking. Sitting in the middle of the continuum (the preferred position) requires more effort, thought and interaction with the patient and their family. Setting the risk thermostat in the middle of the continuum may mean a slightly greater degree of anxiety on the part of the clinician as he/she will need to be more conscious of the possibility of an adverse outcome.

This is shown diagrammatically in Figure 6.3.

In practice, it is more common to veer towards the risk-avoidant end of the continuum as this is driven not just by anxiety, but also high

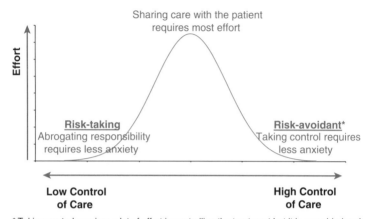

* Taking control requires a lot of effort in controlling the treatment but it is one sided and there is little genuine interaction with the patient. Anxiety settles as control of the situation is taken.

Figure 6.3 **Effort required depending on risk thermostat settings**

workload and limited knowledge base. Clinicians at the risk-taking end of the continuum are more likely to be working in situations where higher levels of risk are dealt with on a daily basis and they become desensitised to the level of risk; for example, crisis teams and inpatient units.

> **Box 6.1 PRACTICE TIP**
>
> If individual clinicians feel or say that they are 'carrying risk' or feel burdened by the risk or say that they 'can't take the risk', it usually means that they are not '*managing* the risk' effectively.

Personal factors that may affect risk management

Most clinicians have learnt to identify and manage the personal factors that may affect risk management although they may be forgotten in the heat of the moment.

Here is a list of *personal* factors in the clinician which may affect the context of risk:

- fear/anxiety and emotional response to the situation
- competence and factual knowledge of clinician:
  - seniority
  - clinician wisdom/experience: 'I don't know how to deal with this'
- mindset of clinician: 'I should be able to save all of my patients'
- workload of clinician:
  - energy/tiredness of clinician
- temperament (empathy, ability to tolerate distress):
  - proximity to the risk
  - experience of patients having a bad outcome.

It is likely that these factors are additive.

Exploring personal factors in more detail

Fear/anxiety and emotional response to risk

Risk is synonymous with danger for many clinicians. If risk is perceived as dangerous, not as something to be assessed and managed with the patient, clinicians are likely to respond as if there is a personal threat. It may be in the form of danger from perceived attack, being stalked or from a fear of loss of registration if a suicide occurs. It is not only danger in the form of physical attack; personality disordered patients intrude on clinicians' feelings and can affect the assessment. However, it would be wrong to ignore the fact that many clinicians are exposed to danger where there is a risk of personal harm. This can occur in many settings. The response to danger is invariably one of fear ('survival anxiety')[4] but there may also be a loss of mental wellbeing from stress. Clinicians may also fear being blamed or fear personal and professional disgrace. If clinicians allow anxiety to affect risk management, it is likely that they will slip into *secondary risk management* (see glossary) which will have a 'corrosive effect on the relationship between the clinician and patient'.[5]

The experience of fear/anxiety promotes an unconscious primitive defence designed to reduce clinician anxiety. The fight or flight response develops in which the patient can become the perceived threat. This is experienced either individually or at a staff group level. Because the defence is designed to protect the clinician as opposed to the patient, it will tend to promote a response of perceiving the patient as being the problem which precludes good risk and clinical management.

Patients can then be blamed (using externally directed hostility)[6] for their problems or treated as consciously creating the problem. For example, 'she's just being manipulative' or 'he's just personality disordered, not mentally ill'. Other common defences are to say, 'it's just a drug-induced psychosis' or 'this patient should be in forensics'. Anxious clinicians cannot reflect on what they are doing which will further reduce capacity for good risk assessment.

The task for individual clinicians and for clinical leaders is to create an environment in which risk assessment and management can occur whilst recognising the reality of risk posed to staff. When clinician anxiety is reduced, this will lead to an increased capacity to see the patient objectively and compassionately. Reduced clinician anxiety also reduces patient anxiety. This leads to better risk management. Clinician anxiety can be used as a tool to help assess the risk and as a tool to create dialogue within the team about risk; that is, using the fear of the clinician in group discussion as a tool to explore the likelihood of the risk occurring.

Competence and factual knowledge of clinician

- Seniority
- Clinician wisdom/experience

Increasing knowledge and experience would normally lead to an assumption that the capacity to manage risk would also be greater. This is usually the case but in those instances where team leaders or clinical leaders (e.g. consultant psychiatrists) are risk-avoidant, their seniority can cause substantial difficulties. Senior clinicians are sometimes risk-avoidant as a result of a patient having a bad outcome and the clinician being keel-hauled in a public setting, such as a coroner's court. The best practice of confidential inquiries, peer review and individual supervision should limit this experience.

Mindset of clinician: 'I should be able to save all of my patients'

To carry this mindset which has been described as an 'over inflated concept of duty of care'[7] is a recipe for burnout and rescuing behaviour on the part of the clinician. Although at times families, coroners and the media expect clinicians to prevent all suicides, this is not possible and the task is not to save all patients but to do the best within the limitations of the individual and the service.

Workload of clinician

- Energy/tiredness of clinician.

This point is self evident but can have a substantial effect on the capacity to manage risk. Making decisions at 3 a.m. is a different experience to making the same decisions at 3 p.m. Clinicians should be mindful of

> ## Box 6.2 PERSONAL RESPONSES TO RISK
>
> **Practice points**
> - If risk is managed by reducing clinician anxiety (secondary risk management), the risk to the patient may increase.
> - If clinician/patient discomfort is reduced indiscriminately, opportunities for learning from and improving the symptoms may also be reduced.
> - 'In order to achieve therapeutic gain, it is sometimes necessary to take risks. A strategy of total risk avoidance can lead to excessively restrictive management, which may in itself be damaging to the individual.'[8]

the affect that their workload and tiredness is having on their decision-making.

Temperament (empathy, ability to tolerate distress)

- Proximity to the risk.
- Experience of patients having a bad outcome.

Within the mental health field, there is a wide variety of sub-specialities. Some clinicians are more able to care for some patients than others and it is important for them to be mindful of any personal characteristics which may affect decision-making in risky situations. Similarly, if clinicians have had a situation where there has been a bad outcome and that has had a substantial impact, consideration needs to be given to how this is affecting risk decision-making.

Finally, for some patients (not psychotic patients), it is often useful to sit with a certain degree of psychological tension as this will be the driver which helps them make necessary changes in their personal lives. It may well be important to support patients in this whilst recognising that both patients and clinicians may sit with a higher degree of risk for a period of time. This will be explored further in the clinical skills section of this book.

Notes

1 Murphy D 2002 Risk assessment as collective clinical judgment. *Criminal Behaviour and Mental Health*, 12:169–78.

2 Undrill G 2007 The risks of risk assessment. *Advances in Psychiatric Treatment*, 13:291–7.

3 Adams J 1995 *Risk*. Routledge Publications, London.

4 Nitsun M 1996 *The Anti-Group. Destructive Forces in the Group and their Creative Potential.* Routledge, London.

5 Undrill, above, n 2.

6 Murphy, above, n 1.

7 Carroll A 2007 Are violence risk assessment tools clinically useful? *Australian and New Zealand Journal of Psychiatry*, 41:301–7

8 New Zealand Ministry of Health 1998 Guidelines for Clinical Risk Assessment and Management in Mental Health Services. New Zealand Ministry of Health.

7 Systemic aspects of risk assessment and management

Risk is never limited to the patient. Clinicians, family, the wider community, other health services and so on will all be involved. At its simplest level, risk will be managed between one individual clinician and the patient but this is an unusual situation. More commonly the potential consequences of an adverse outcome will be felt by a much wider selection of people and they are likely to become involved in some way in the assessment and management of the risk. Family and friends are often vital informants who will help identify early warning signs and triggers for risk behaviours.

Multidisciplinary team (MDT) dynamics affecting risk assessment and management

Group cohesiveness

Within a mental health team, there is likely to be more than one clinician involved in the care of a patient and even if there is only one clinician directly involved, the patient's care will be discussed in a MDT format. The cohesiveness or otherwise of the staff group can have a large bearing on risk management. Group cohesiveness can break down for several different reasons, such as weak leadership or one clinician holding a grudge against another. Any psychological process affecting an individual clinician can also affect the MDT as a group. As is the case with individual staff, the capacity of the group to think and reflect may be impaired in a setting of risk and perceived danger.[1]

For example, if the psychiatric registrar is anxious about the care of the patient, this may make other clinicians anxious and the whole team becomes risk-avoidant. This will then need to be managed as a team problem. Conversely, if the MDT is supportive, anxiety will be lower and the risk thermostat for the team will be set differently.

Another influence on group decision-making is the concept of 'groupthink'.[2, 3] Groupthink is a type of thought exhibited by group members who try to minimise conflict and reach consensus without critically testing, analysing and evaluating ideas. Individual creativity, uniqueness and independent thinking are lost in the pursuit of group cohesiveness. During groupthink, members of the group avoid promoting viewpoints outside the comfort zone of consensus thinking. Groupthink may cause groups to make hasty, irrational decisions where individual doubts are set aside for fear of upsetting the group's balance. Groupthink is more likely to occur in situations in which there is directive leadership, the group perceive themselves as being under stress from external threats or where there are excessive difficulties in the decision-making tasks. Moral dilemmas are also likely to invoke groupthink.

Difficult risk decisions often have to be made when a group feels threatened or when there are moral dilemmas. Groupthink should be considered if risk management in the MDT is problematic. It is likely that groupthink occurs not infrequently in MDT settings and should be considered as a cause of poor decision-making even when the MDT feels cohesive.

Clinicians as custodians

Inpatient mental health services are often given the task of being custodians of patients and ensuring that they cannot leave. The conflict between being custodial and trying to be therapeutic at the same time can create tension and anxiety which may challenge group cohesiveness. It is possible for the requirements of custodial care to become paramount in the minds of staff and when this occurs, a power differential will be created in which therapeutic relationships cannot occur. The capacity to explore risk issues with patients is then substantially decreased and any information which is gathered may well be compromised by the power differential which is present.

Clinicians perceiving patients as hostile

When some clinicians perceive a patient as being hostile and 'negative' and other clinicians perceive the same patient as being helpless and a victim of their circumstances, tension will be set up within the staff group. This is sometimes diagnosed as the patient 'splitting', which may be correct; for example, 'the manipulative patient', but any tension or conflict within the staff group needs to be recognised as well. The classical scenario is of an inpatient who 'threatens' to self-harm on the ward. It is not unusual for some clinicians to feel that the patient is fully in control of their actions and to say that they are just manipulating the situation to get attention, and for other clinicians to say that the patient can't help their feelings. In these situations, risk assessment can be sabotaged by dissenting clinicians.

A more problematic scenario is one in which there is group solidarity against one particular patient who becomes the perceived enemy. In some units, there may be subtle processes set up to avoid admitting new patients, thereby avoiding the risk. If there are clinicians who want to admit the patient, they may well be ostracised and group cohesiveness goes out the window.

It almost goes without saying that the team leader needs to have good skills in risk assessment and management in order to not to have to rely on his/her authority. Being able to model best practice and create a climate in which risk assessment is seen as being core business is vital.[4]

- Does the team have processes in place to manage group anxiety?
- Does the team make decisions depending on the greatest anxiety of any individual team member or does the team leader have the capacity to manage stress and implement good risk assessment and management processes?
- Is the team caught up in mindless completion of forms rather than being able to explore the risk issues?
- Does form-filling become a defence to protect the anxiety of the team?

All of these questions should be in the mind of the team leader and there should be sufficient time for the team to reflect on these issues.

In summary, utilising collective judgment is likely to improve the quality of the risk assessment as long as the 'collective judgment' is not distorted by pathological processes working within the group.[5]

See Murphy's *Risk Assessment As Collective Clinical Judgment* (2002)[6] for a more detailed discussion of this topic.

Exercise 1 — level of risk changing over time

Alison is 45 years old and is suffering from a major depressive disorder with current suicidal intent. She has made one attempt at suicide in the past. Her treatment for previous episodes of depression has included hospitalisation, ECT and prophylactic antidepressants. Her very supportive family is coming to the end of their capacity to cope with her suicidal depression and asks for your help. You want to admit her to

---

BOX 7.1 SYSTEMIC ASPECTS OF RISK

Practice points
- Risk is not limited to one person. There are invariably systemic components to it.
- Family are vital informants in the assessment and management of risk.
- The patient, family and MDT should consider the risk.
- Adverse outcomes can be prepared for by the patient, family and MDT.
- Team leaders have a vital role to play in managing both individual staff and team anxiety. Any evidence of secondary risk management should lead to a review of individual, team or wider system functioning.
- The team should not succumb to the greatest anxiety of any one member of the treatment team (e.g. case manager, psychiatrist or team leader).
- As with individual clinicians, the MDT need time to reflect on their actions.

---

hospital because you feel that her suicidal intent is acute. You know that if you admit her to hospital, she will be taking the last available bed and this is the beginning of the weekend.

As you read this, consider where your risk thermostat is set. What are the factors that have influenced its setting? Identify the systemic components which may affect your risk management. Possible answers to this exercise appear in Appendix 3.

(The management of these issues will be covered in Part 2.)

Other systemic issues which will have a bearing on risk assessment and management include:

- Resources available. Do individual clinicians or the team feel that there are often insufficient resources available to manage certain situations? How is this managed? (See Page 116.)
- Health and safety processes; for example, are there alarm buttons in the offices?
- Having a risk management team who give feedback.
- The availability of guidelines. Are these available in printed form at each base?
- Being aware of the increased risk which occurs during shift change in inpatient units is something which all staff should carry in the back of their minds.

BOX 7.2 PRACTICE TIP

- Clinicians can ask for advice from colleagues and senior clinical staff within and outside the team and make use of MDT reviews.
- Case conferences are an excellent way of exploring risk and treatment possibilities.
- Consider requesting a second opinion or a consultation from a specialist service such as the forensic service or the regional personality disorder service or using other expert practitioners.
- The legal services of the mental health service are available for advice in unusual circumstances.
- Refer to the guidelines and other resources listed on pages 4–5.

Some of the bullet points above are related to organisational issues and are beyond the direct influence of individual clinicians. Nonetheless, it is important to recognise the influences which these systemic issues may have on risk management of individual or groups of patients. Part 4, advanced skills, explores some of the organisational issues and is primarily written for senior clinical staff. For individual clinicians, however, it is vital to remember to include others (not least the patient and their families) in the assessment and management of risk and not to feel that there is no-one else involved in the management of it. Remember, nearly all clinicians work in a team and have many other resources available to assist in developing and implementing risk management and treatment plans.

BOX 7.3 CLINICAL TIP: REQUESTING A SECOND OPINION

- Requesting a second opinion is an excellent way of receiving support, having a fresh set of eyes look over the problem and getting specialist advice.
- Clinicians will get far greater benefit from this resource if they:
  - make their best effort of doing the risk assessment first and not expect the specialist to do it all for them
  - outline clearly the questions that they would like assistance with. This is more likely to lead to a collegial response which will have a teaching component to it as well.

Notes

1 Murphy D 2002 Risk assessment as collective clinical judgment. *Criminal Behaviour and Mental Health*, 12:169–78.

2 Janis IL 1982 *Groupthink: Psychological Studies of Policy Decisions and Fiascos*, Houghton Mifflin Harcourt International Publishers, Illinois.

3 Schafer M, Crichlow S 1996 Antecedents of groupthink: a quantitative study. *The Journal of Conflict Resolution*, 40(3), Sept:415–35.

4 Murphy, above, n 1.

5 Murphy, above, n 1.

6 Murphy, above, n 1.

PART 2

CLINICAL SKILLS TRAINING

8 Approaches to risk assessment 1

> Risk assessment is not a new technique, although the emphasis is different. It requires no more and no less than a full clinical history and examination.[1]

As can be seen from the quotation, risk assessment is nothing new. It starts from the first contact that a clinician has with the patient and continues every time the patient is seen until discharge. Risk assessment allows clinicians to paint a picture of where the risk for the patient lies within the context of their illness and their environment. It helps in planning management of both the illness and risk behaviours.

In the general clinical setting, screening, assessment and management of risk will all be occurring simultaneously. Often, the assessment process will be therapeutic in its own right and becomes management. Often, after talking about their suicidal preoccupation, patients say, 'I'm feeling better now that I've told you that. I was scared to let anybody know how I really felt.'

The chapters on clinical skills are written in such a way that an assumption may be made that each skill can be separated out in the clinical situation and applied incrementally. The presentation of risk assessment and management as separate clinical skills is artificial and not intended to reflect clinical practice. The skills and exercises in successive chapters build on those practised in the previous chapters.

The process of risk assessment also allows for the development of rapport with the patient and should always be seen as a component of treatment, not just an exercise undertaken to fulfil bureaucratic requirements. As is increasingly the case with all clinical work, there should be an expectation that documentation will be shared with the patient. *Every time* the patient is seen, there should be an assessment for the imminence and previously identified patterns of risk. On an inpatient ward, this may happen every few minutes, whilst in an outpatient setting, it may only occur every 3–6 months when a stable patient is reviewed.

It is a process of combining the 'here and now' assessment with the knowledge of the patient's past to try and predict the future. The 'here and now' assessment will include the patient's mental state, the patient's current circumstances, systemic issues including resources available, geographical factors and consideration of the clinician's own response to the situation.

The stages of risk assessment/management do not change and are fairly straightforward: screen for whether the risk exists or not, assess the seriousness and imminence, assess the risk factors and address them. Risk assessment is an evolutionary process, not an outcome. It allows a group of clinicians to defend the defensible by documenting the systematic assessment of an individual. As clinicians become more knowledgeable about a patient, they can add more information about the risk factors and the function of the risk. As some risk is inherent for all patients in one form or another, clinicians should constantly be thinking about possible risks. If the full clinical assessment has been done adequately, the risk assessment should develop more easily.

A full clinical history depends on other sources of information as well as the history from the patient. Risk assessment is no different. This includes accounts from relatives and other informants. In practice, the general mental health worker will often have concerns raised by family and friends and these concerns will be used in conjunction with the clinical assessment. Family or friends who live with a patient are often the first to notice problems.

The other vital component of risk assessment is knowledge of risk factors known to increase the likelihood of the risk behaviour. Access to standardised lists of risk factors is a requirement for good risk assessment. See pages 80–81 and 84–85 for examples.

Risk assessment does have a predictive quality to it but primarily because of the dynamic factors, it can never be 100% accurate. Risk prediction tends to be more accurate in the short-term. As with routine clinical practice, when there is uncertainty, taking advice from colleagues or asking for second opinions or discussing it in the MDT meeting is good practice.

The process of risk assessment can be very quick and easy with some patients where the risk is felt to be minimal, whereas for other patients risk assessment and management turns into a very detailed undertaking making use of specialised assessment tools and may occur over a protracted period of time. This tiered approach[2] of basic assessment at one end of a continuum to extremely detailed assessment at the other end will be well known to most clinicians and has been advocated as best practice in the UK. Depending on the level of detail required, the documentation will be quite varied.

This book does not cover clinical skills about how to ask specific questions relating to the risk of suicide or violence. These skills are covered in detail in some guidelines for suicide and violence and in books on clinical skills, and should be taught to all clinicians during their training.

Types of risk assessment

There are four major approaches to risk assessment but there is overlap within each.

1 unaided clinical judgment
2 using actuarial tools
3 using a psychodynamic contribution
4 structured clinical judgment.

Unaided clinical judgment

Unaided clinical judgment is exactly what it says. A history is taken, personality functioning is described, the mental state examined and demographic factors considered. Although unaided clinical judgment has importance, it has low inter-rater reliability and relatively low predictive value. A further problem with unaided clinical judgment is that it is also quite vulnerable to heuristic biases. Unaided clinical judgment is not recommended currently. For risk assessment of severe violence, a government committee in Scotland has stated that unaided clinical judgment cannot continue to be supported.[3]

Actuarial tools

Actuarial tools were primarily developed for research purposes rather than for clinical practice and so they do not always meet the needs of everyday situations. Actuarial risk assessment tools have also been criticised as being less sensitive than clinical risk assessment to individual differences since actuarial tools on specific risks are developed from data on large populations and are therefore not specific to the individual person.

> Actuarial risk tools do not inform clinicians about the circumstances, severity or imminence of the act in question. Another, more crucial problem is the inability of this approach to take into account fluctuations in the level of risk as circumstances change.[4]

However, an actuarial statistical approach to risk assessment can enhance the predictions based on clinical assessments and can communicate the degree of risk in qualitative terms. Actuarial tools do have their place in that factors known to be of relevance for the risk being assessed — for example, criminal history, substance abuse, impulsivity and marital status — can be rated for their presence or not. Actuarial scales tend to focus on static risk factors, less on the dynamic ones. It is the dynamic factors which make the job of risk prediction so difficult for mental health professionals compared to other branches of medicine where there are often fewer changing variables. Actuarial data and standardised assessment tools should inform the risk assessment, not substitute for it. In recent years, standardised scales have increasingly included items for dynamic factors and treatment issues. With this shift, the use of standardised scales which focused only on static factors is lessening.

Standardised scales are discussed further in Chapter 18.

Psychodynamic contribution

A psychodynamic contribution can add important information. The understanding of the risk behaviour for a patient can be enhanced using psychodynamic principles. For example, a violent patient may only attack other men of a certain age because they remind the patient of his father, or a patient with PTSD may only become suicidal on the anniversary of a violent assault. Further useful information may be elicited from feelings that the patient has towards different clinicians and the responses of clinicians towards the patient. Psychodynamic principles used in risk assessment are discussed further in Chapter 16.

Structured clinical judgment (SCJ)

The unaided clinical versus actuarial debate has led to the development of risk prediction instruments which adopt a combined approach and recognise the importance of both static (and dynamic) actuarial variables and the clinical/risk management items that clinicians normally take into account in risk assessments of individuals. The combined approach is called structured clinical judgment (SCJ) and represents a composite of empirical knowledge and clinical/professional expertise. Structured risk assessments act as *aides-memoire* and make sure that all relevant information is collected.[5]

Structured clinical judgment is a process which blends structured assessment of risk factors with clinical judgment, including the identification of the patterns of risk behaviours. On top of the usual history and mental state examination, the static and dynamic factors *known to be of empirical relevance* in the context of the patient's illness are identified. This is then put together into a plan which addresses the risks. Structured clinical judgment is currently the recommended baseline modality of assessment. If the risk assessment is completed using a structured format, communication will be enhanced and be more transparent as the documentation will be clearly laid out and easily read. If all clinicians in a service use the same format, individual biases and personal opinions are less likely to intrude on the process.

Several structured instruments have been developed to assess risk in clinical contexts. These include the Historical/Clinical/Risk Management 20-item (HCR-20) scale[6] for assessing violence and more recently a scale for the assessment of suicide risk developed by Bouch.[7] These structured instruments are discussed in more detail in Chapter 18.

Advantages and disadvantages of SCJ using standardised rating scales

A difficulty with the use of structured instruments which include standardised rating scales is that best practice recommends they be validated. Unfortunately, for the general clinician seeing a wide variety of patients with differing risks, there is no one instrument which is currently available which has been validated. As yet, the literature has only generated one standardised assessment tool (the START)[8] which attempts to cover a wide variety of risks, albeit with a rather thin evidence base currently. This is perhaps not surprising given the focus of research (mostly from forensic services) which tends to be on specific risks and the development of tools to help identify each risk.

Most rating scales require specific training which tends only to occur for staff in forensic settings and a few clinicians in general settings. Using rating scales also takes time which is often a hindrance to compliance with documentation for clinicians.

> If the tools are not used in a way that demonstrably adds something to standard clinical processes, then the time expended on paperwork will inevitably detract from the efficiency of service provision.[9]

Given this, it is perhaps not surprising that 'locally developed, unstandardised, unvalidated schemes are often used in preference to standardised tools with demonstrated validity'.[10]

For the busy general clinician, risk assessment on a day-to-day basis may vary from assessment of violence with one patient to assessment of suicidality in the next and then to assessment of self-harm or assessment of harm from others. To utilise different standardised assessment tools for each of these patients when the risk may well turn out to be of minor significance would be pragmatically impossible and clinicians might be justified in complaining that the standardised assessment tools are too unwieldy. As Carroll (2007) comments when discussing the difficulties for general clinicians using standardised rating scales:

> … to secure a lasting rapprochement between the academic and clinical spheres, new ways of embedding risk assessment technology into everyday practice are required.[11]

To compound matters even further, the initial documentation of risk may well vary depending on whether the first assessment occurs in an acute setting or takes place in the context of a routine 'cold' assessment. In the acute assessment, the level of risk is likely to be much higher with the emphasis being on the here and now. Documentation in this setting may be limited to an identification of the risk with basic information about risk factors. More information will be gathered about risk factors once the immediate risk has been contained. For the routine assessment, the level of risk is likely to be lower and the emphasis will be on identification of risk factors which will need to be considered when the patient presents in the future.

In both these settings, the likelihood is that the risk assessment will not be completed during the initial meeting with the patient but will become an evolutionary process with more information added to it as the patient becomes better known. In forensic settings, the risk behaviour has usually occurred already. The patient will have been incarcerated in prison or admitted to hospital and the risk assessment can occur over a period of time. The focus is often on prediction of future episodes as well as prevention.

A pragmatic compromise for the general mental health clinician

The dilemma of how clinicians can practice SCJ has been considered carefully in the UK and best practice recommendations are, currently, that locally developed forms 'should be designed with evidence-based principles in mind, stating clear and verifiable risk indicators'.[12] This is a compromise allowing general clinicians to practise well without being encumbered with time consuming specialised rating scales. For the general mental health clinician:

> the initial risk assessment exercise should consist of a structured process of more or less standard questions aimed at eliciting factors increasing the risk (and which will reflect the evidence base around the risk) and which assists clinical judgment. It could be called an *aide-memoire* or a framework. After the clinician addresses these standard questions,

it will be possible to determine whether a more in-depth assessment is needed using existing, evidenced-based toolkits for the particular population.[13]

The risk assessment and management model (hereafter referred to as simply 'the model') used for the exercises in this book is a structured format for assessing, documenting and managing the risk while making use of the static and dynamic risk factors known to be associated with the type of risk being assessed. It is important to have an *empirically validated list of risk factors* available for common risks such as violence or suicide and these can be found on pages 80–81 and 84–85. This is then combined with the clinician's knowledge of the patient and, importantly, the patient's own perspective.

The major function of the model is as a 'decision support tool'[14] designed to assist the general clinician manage risk within the context of the illness. The framework incorporates the basic structures of standardised tools: focus on known static, dynamic and protective risk factors as well as a focus on management. The lists of empirical risk factors for each type of risk are separate to the model and can be updated as new research is published. The model is both an assessment and management tool and attempts to meet the following requirements:

- it has to be useful for clinicians and patients and facilitate clinical practice[15]
- it should not require too much in the way of training
- it should be short enough to be able to be completed on a regular basis by all mental health clinicians
- where possible, the document should be completed with the input of the patient and the final version should also be given to the patient (and family as appropriate)
- it should blend in with treatment documentation.

In practice, the model is easily applied and is sufficient for most situations and may lay the foundation for the administration of a standardised tool if required.

- The model prompts for clinical information to help identify patterns of risk and to understand the function of the risk behaviour.
- The model focuses on static and dynamic factors and generates early warning signs, relapse indicators and proposes management for the risk within the context of the illness.
- The format is structured ensuring that all clinicians follow the same process no matter what the risk, and it covers the major areas of risk assessment.

- The model is a series of questions with prompts that are designed to focus the attention of the clinician on the key areas of risk assessment and management.
- When combined with a treatment plan which also focuses on early warning signs, triggers and relapse indicators, many of the items generated from the model can be 'cut and pasted' into the treatment plan.
- Because the model used is not a standardised rating scale, it only provides prompts for risk factors which may be relevant for each particular risk.
- By not having tick boxes for risk factors included in the risk assessment and management form (Figure 8.1), *critical risk factors* tend to be automatically identified as clinicians limit their focus to what is most important for their patient.

This model has changed many times over 6 years, has been refined and field tested in a mental health service of over 500 clinicians, and will continue to evolve. Feedback from a variety of sectors including Emergency Departments (EDs), general practitioners and crisis mental health teams has been of central importance in its continuing development. A major requirement in the development of this model has been the need to ensure that it integrates well with assessment and treatment documentation. It also needs to work within a tiered approach to risk.[16] Documentation on risk within the clinical assessment can be 'cut and pasted' into this model. In a similar fashion the recommendations for interventions identified in this model can be cut and pasted into the treatment plan.

The model is weighted towards prevention and helping a clinician, who does not know the patient, manage an acute situation. In general mental health services this may be of more practical relevance. It avoids statements about level of risk. This is less common in tools derived from forensic services where the emphasis is more likely to be on prediction, level of risk and prevention in the longer term. The section of the model focussing on the function of the risk behaviour could be criticised for assuming that all risk behaviour is driven by frustration but in practice this is not always the case as it can also be coldly goal-directed and sometimes occurs in order to obtain a response from others — secondary gain. When this section has been left out of previous versions, the planning for possible interventions to manage frustration or secondary gain has often been forgotten to the detriment of the care of the patient. This section is sometimes very useful in picking up 'signature risk signs' specific to the patient; for example, a patient who has increased risk at the time of an anniversary.

In general mental health settings one of the most common risks identified is the *risk of relapse*. Risk of relapse is not usually considered to be a 'risk' within the risk literature. It is normally addressed within a treatment plan but the process for assessment and management is identical to that of routine risk management. Identification of dynamic risk factors, consideration of static factors which increase the propensity for relapse, and identification of early warning signs and triggers are no different. Because risk of relapse is also a risk factor for suicide, violence and so on, management of the risk of relapse is always required. The model can be utilised to identify the factors of importance for relapse prevention even when no other risks are identified. In practice, it is rare for relapse management not to be incorporated as an integral component of the risk management.

The completed form will generate interventions to be implemented in the longer term but the assessment of the level of risk in the acute/crisis setting remains the responsibility of the clinician on the spot. It gives the clinician guidance and a head start into what interventions may help but the decision about which interventions to utilise is left to the clinician and patient at the time.

If the risk documentation takes a structured narrative form, this allows the focus of inquiry to be directed and also allows risk factors to be contextualised and patterns identified.[17] As a result, tick boxes have been excluded. The model allows for the level of risk to change over time and does not need updating with fluctuations of the clinical condition. If the risk plan is included in the overall treatment plan, it should not undermine in any way the overall thrust of treatment. (The treatment plan should include management of the identified dynamic risk factors.)

Examples of completed risk assessments/plans are in Appendix 3.

Static factors on risk assessment/plans

Most risk assessment/plans in general psychiatry do not document *all* the static factors. The model prompts for the major static risk factors only. If clinicians are developing a complete risk management plan for a patient — for example, a patient in a forensic unit with a risk of violence who is close to discharge — the risk management plan might include a detailed list of all the static risk factors of importance, especially psychopathy, and will describe the influence of the static factors on the current risk. The decision whether to document the static risk factors separately will vary from patient to patient. On the one hand, it is always useful to be able to see the static risk factors separately but on the other hand imposing this on staff means yet more filling out of forms and makes compliance less likely. Also, 'forms irritate the people who have to fill them in'.[18] The important point is to be able to use the static factors to help inform the management of the patient in the longer term.

When developing the prompts for interventions, it is tempting to be prescriptive to ensure that all bases are covered. For example, the following prompts cover most situations:

- social interventions
- medical interventions
- client-centred interventions
- admission to inpatient units or crisis respite, etc.

When headings like those above are used on risk forms, it is implied that each section needs to be filled out and clinicians are tempted to write an intervention for each prompt such as: 'Take medication' or 'Go to crisis respite' and other self-evident options.

If history was completely predictive then interventions could be presented in a decision tree. A vital task when developing forms is to encourage clinicians to step outside the triage, diagnose and treatment process for risk management and support the patient by getting to know them. Find out what moves the patient, what and who influences them and then present a resource for working with them through a crisis where risk is elevated.

A resource that is prescriptive is potentially less reliable, but a resource that provides insight and information to the clinician on the spot supports interventions that can reduce the likelihood of the risk behaviour occurring.

Figure 8.1 is the complete model with commentary inserted into the boxes (in italics) where clinical information would usually be written. Many of the prompts have been taken from actuarial information. As clinicians get used to the format of the documentation, the prompts can be left out, which simplifies the form somewhat. When electronic health records are used, the prompts can be made to automatically disappear from the finished form. The form has been kept down to two A4 pages as anything longer than this seems to reduce the likelihood of clinicians completing it. When using this form, validated scales for the relevant risk should be utilised for reference.

The model, as printed over the next two pages, appears not to give sufficient room for information to be adequately documented. If there is more than one risk or if there have been several episodes of the risk behaviour previously, there would not be enough room in a hard copy

BOX 8.1 PRACTICE TIPS

- Whilst not semantically correct, clinicians seem to prefer the phrases which use the word 'risk' rather than the more correct phrase 'adverse outcomes'.
- The box for previous episodes of the risks is frequently not big enough when the risk is that of violence or self-harm. When this form is used in an electronic version, the box expands accordingly.
- When used in an electronic health record, the right-hand column used for interventions usually disappears and becomes another horizontal row in the form. Some clinicians prefer to use the version with the interventions opposite the risk factors.
- Being able to cut and paste interventions from the risk management plan into a treatment plan is very useful.

version of this form. However, most clinicians utilise this documentation from a Microsoft Word template, or similar. The template can be copied into a separate patient file and information keyed directly into the template.

RISK ASSESSMENT AND MANAGEMENT FORM

DATE OF PLAN		NAME OF PATIENT	Place label here
EXPIRY DATE (maximum — 6 months)	Always complete this to ensure a review.	Surname: DOB:	Given name: Patient number:

CURRENT DIAGNOSES AND CLINICAL CONCERNS Include personality traits/disorder.

This segment sets the scene for the rest of the form. It puts the subsequent description of risk firmly into the context of the patient's illness.

CURRENT RISKS What is/are the risk/s? Who is the risk to, what means might be used and where might it happen?

This segment is self evident. Be as specific as possible. If the risk identified is a risk of relapse of illness, this can be a useful place to document it. The rest of the form will help prompt for early warning signs (EWS), triggers and relapse indicators.

PREVIOUS EPISODES OF THE RISK(S) Where did it happen, to whom and when? What was the context — illness, situational factors, substance use, not taking medications? Document each episode in as much detail as possible. Identify recurring patterns (risk scenarios) from this information.

This box is vitally important. A good description of previous episodes of risk behaviour, and the circumstances in which it happened will identify patterns which are likely to be repeated in the future. Did the risk behaviour occur during an episode of illness? If so what was happening in the patient's life at that time? Where possible, identify patterns and EWS which will help predict future episodes. See page 33.

WHAT ARE THE FUNCTIONS OF THE RISK BEHAVIOURS? For example, acting on delusions or hallucinations; self-harm reducing tension or distress; violence or threats being effective, etc.	**WHAT INTERVENTIONS HELP ADDRESS THESE FACTORS? WHAT SKILLS ARE BEING DEVELOPED TO DO THIS?** For example, reality orientation; self-soothing; cognitive skills; dialectical behaviour therapy (DBT) skills; etc.
Developing an understanding of the reasons for the risk behaviour occurring will help the patient develop insight and thus be more likely to participate in their management. It brings the focus back to the illness and reduces the tendency by clinicians to blame. For some risk behaviours, management cannot move forward until a hypothesis for the motivation, meaning or purpose for the risk behaviour has been developed; for example, self-harming behaviour. This segment may be easier to complete once the dynamic risk factors have been identified but is included higher up in the form because of its importance.	This column is where risk assessment becomes risk management. This box and the succeeding boxes in the right-hand columns can be 'cut and pasted' to the treatment plan. Developing interventions requires close collaboration with the patient, and sensitivity.

Figure 8.1 Risk assessment and management form

WHAT IN THIS PERSON'S HISTORY CONTRIBUTES TO INCREASING RISK?
For example, history of substance use; conduct disorder; impulsivity; etc. Use the validated scales from your training manual.

This is an exploration of the static factors and should give some guidance for how close the patient is likely to be to the tipping point as a result of their past experiences.

WHAT MENTAL STATE FACTORS INCREASE THESE RISKS? For example, hallucinations, delusions, feelings of rejection, depression, etc.	**WHAT INTERVENTIONS HELP ADDRESS THESE FACTORS?** For example, compliance with medication, reduced stress.
Once again, this brings the risk back into the context of the patient's illness.	As is the case for everything in the right-hand columns, it is virtually impossible to complete these boxes without close cooperation with the patient.
Identify early warning signs and triggers of these factors. Who notices the changes first?	
This is the first opportunity to explore drivers for the mental state factors. This segment is likely to be copied straight into the patient's treatment plan.	
WHAT EXTERNAL, ENVIRONMENTAL OR SITUATIONAL FACTORS AFFECT THE RISK? For example, substance use, living conditions, relationship problems, not taking medication, etc.	**WHAT INTERVENTIONS HELP ADDRESS THESE FACTORS?** For example, respite, reducing drug use, phoning a friend.
Expressions of the risk behaviour are more likely to occur in certain situations; for example, home, when drunk, after arguments. Being mindful of these will be important in developing interventions.	
WHAT SKILLS OR RESOURCES ARE THE PROTECTIVE FACTORS? For example, insight into illness, supportive family, stable accommodation, compliance with medication, etc.	**WHO ELSE IS INVOLVED IN THE CARE AND TREATMENT OF THIS PATIENT?** For example, family, friends, etc.
Utilising protective factors in treatment is obvious but the documentation of them is also therapeutic. Patients and their families take comfort from seeing protective factors put down on paper.	This is a reminder of the systemic responsibility which can be taken for the risk as well as being a reminder for the after-hours clinician to use other resources for help.

TEAMS AND CLINICIANS INVOLVED

THIS FORM MUST INCLUDE A FACE SHEET and TREATMENT PLAN

COMPULSORY COPY TO: Crisis Team
ALSO COPIED TO: ☐ Patient   ☐ Family   ☐ GP   ☐ Emergency Department

☐ Accommodation provider   ☐ Other (specify)

PRINT NAME AND DESIGNATION	Date	Time

Have you put enough information in this form to help a colleague treat and care for this patient in an emergency?

Figure 8.1, Cont'd

Notes

1 Maden A 1996 Risk assessment in psychiatry. *British Journal of Hospital Medicine*, 56(2/3).

2 Royal College of Psychiatrists 2008 Rethinking Risk to Others in Mental Health Services. Final report of a scoping group. June 2008 Royal College of Psychiatrists College Report CR 150, June, p 38.

3 Scottish Executive 2000. *Report of the Committee on Serious, Violent and Sexual Offenders*. Scottish Executive, Edinburgh.

4 Bouch J, Marshall JJ 2005 Suicide risk: structured professional judgment. *Advances in Psychiatric Treatment*, 11:84–91.

5 Maden A 2003 Standardised risk assessment: why all the fuss? *Psychiatric Bulletin*, 27,201–4.

6 Webster C D, Douglas KF, Eaves D et al 1997 *HCR-20: Assessing Risk of Violence* (version 2). Mental Health Law and Policy Institute, Simon Fraser University, Vancouver.

7 Bouch & Marshall, above, n 4.

8 Webster CD, Nicholls TL, Martin ML, Desmarais SL, Brink J 2006 Short-Term Assessment of Risk and Treatability (START): The case for a New Structured Professional Judgment Scheme. *Behavioural Science and the Law*, 24:747–66.

9 Carroll A 2007 Are violence risk assessment tools clinically useful? *Australian and New Zealand Journal of Psychiatry*, 41:301–7.

10 Higgins N, Watts D, Bindman J, Slade M, Thonicroft G 2005 Assessing violence risk in general adult psychiatry. *Psychiatric Bulletin*, 29:131–3.

11 Carroll, above, n 9.

12 Department of Health UK 2007 Best Practice in Managing Risk. Principles and Evidence for Best Practice in the Assessment and Management of Risk to Self and Others in Mental Health Services. Document prepared for the National Mental Health Risk Management Programme, June 2007.

13 Royal College of Psychiatrists, above, n 2.

14 McNeil D, Gregory AL, Lam JN, Binder RL, Sullivan GR 2003 Utility of decision support tools for assessing acute risk of violence. *Journal Consult Clin Psychol*, 71:945–53.

15 Royal College of Psychiatrists, above, n 2, Mullen, p 37.

16 Royal College of Psychiatrists, above, n 2, p 38.

17 Higgins et al, above, n 10.

18 Maden, above, n 5.

9 Approaches to risk assessment 2

Risk assessment is best described in terms of human endeavour, not in the language of scientific measurement.[1]

Screening for risk

Screening for risk is a routine part of all assessments. Screening for suicide risk will be used as the example to describe the process. The assessment of suicidal risk is one of the most common and basic procedures in psychiatry.[2] It is probably the purest example of a risk assessment as the process requires close interaction with the patient, is incremental in that the next question is based on the response to the previous question, and interventions will be based on both treating the underlying illness and preventing the risk behaviour from occurring.

Unless the patient spontaneously comments that they are considering suicide, the clinician will need to prompt for it. An index of suspicion should be present for any patient with mood symptoms. If the primary problem is another problem such as psychosis, the mood symptoms may be hidden but the screening questions should still be asked. The first screening question may lead on to an in-depth assessment of the risk or may be sufficient to allow the clinician to determine that the current risk is negligible or absent.

After working towards the questions about suicidality with a question such as, 'How bad have things been?', it will be possible to move on to an initial screening question such as, 'Have you ever felt that life is no longer worth it?' or 'Have you ever felt that you can't carry on?'.

If the verbal and/or non-verbal response to these opening questions is positive, the clinician will then continue to ask more probing questions until the extent of the preoccupation with suicide is apparent. From there, in conjunction with the rest of the assessment, management decisions will be made. For suicide,

BOX 9.1 CLINICAL TIP

(When asking the initial screening questions for risk to self or others, the good clinician will be looking for incongruity between the verbal and non-verbal responses. For example, the non-verbal response of averted eyes, or shifting in the chair should be a prompt for further exploration either later on in the interview or in the near future, depending on the situation.)

because of the acuity which may be present, it is not uncommon for a full assessment to be conducted during the first meeting to determine the level of risk. This is less likely to be the case for violence where the focus is more often on preventing future episodes.

Suicide assessment is incorporated into the body of the clinical assessment. For other risks such as violence and self-harm the process is the same but the index of suspicion may not be as high on the part of the clinician. Suicide is an easily recognised complication of mood disorders whilst other risks such as violence and sexual predation are more likely to be hidden; there may be more shame or a fear that disclosure will be punished in some way, such as incarceration. Violence may be a complication of several different disease processes and may occur even when there is no disease process. A clinician should, however, always include a basic screening for violence. Sexual predation is unlikely to be part of routine general mental health screening unless an index of suspicion is raised in the assessment.

Static factors in the history which make the propensity for violence greater should be considered. These should emerge during the routine questioning of the childhood and personality development. The patient's response to dynamic factors should be explored. A classical example would be an exploration of the patient's likelihood of acting on command hallucinations.

When there is uncertainty about how detailed the risk assessment should be, the rule of thumb should be — do a complete assessment.

The negatives if the risk is minimal will make the process quick, the discovery of positives and consideration of interventions makes it worthwhile.[3]

There are screening tools available (one is included in Chapter 15, risk of violence) but a useful rule of thumb is to consider a more detailed assessment if:

- there are substantive risk issues
- the patient is likely to require treatment after hours
- the patient is likely to make contact with the service in between appointments
- the patient is admitted for treatment to either a respite facility or hospital
- there is a past history of violence, self-harm or suicide attempts.

The decision about the level of detail required within the assessment will also be based on the following question; 'What is the likelihood and imminence of the risk behaviour occurring and what will the consequences be if it occurs?'

As the patient becomes better known and treatment continues, the assessment of the risk will continue alongside the continuing assessment of the patient's clinical condition.

BOX 9.2 CLINICAL TIP
OBSESSIVE-COMPULSIVE DISORDER (OCD)[4]

Learning points:
- Obsessional ruminations are often misinterpreted as indicating risk. There are no recorded cases of a person with OCD carrying out their obsession. By definition, such intrusions are unacceptable and ego-dystonic.
- Risk in OCD is usually related to the consequences of acting on compulsions and urges in order to avoid the anxiety-provoking situations; for example, harm from washing hands too frequently, harm from compulsive hoarding.
- Risk to others may occur when well-meaning attempts are made to prevent compulsive behaviours being carried out.
- Secondary co-morbid illnesses such as depression, which is driven by the distress of the OCD, may create risk of suicide and should be assessed.

Assessment and documentation exercise

The first exercise in this section starts the process of assessing and documenting risk. Often, the first presentation is a phone call or an assessment in the Emergency Department (ED). Information may be limited but a start needs to be made. The initial identification of the risk may also create anxiety on the part of the clinician. The process of simply documenting what is known creates a degree of objectivity which will immediately reduce anxiety. The purpose of the following exercise is to simply practise documenting identified risk and consider to whom, when, where and what means might be used. Practising the exercises will give you an opportunity to get used to the routine questions which are central to any risk assessment. With practice, there will be increasing familiarity which is a risk management skill in its own right. Familiarity with the process can reduce risk by a factor of 17.[5]

For each of the examples below answer the following questions.

1 What are the risks?
2 Whom is the risk to?
3 When may it happen?
4 Where may it happen?
5 What means might be used?

Try and write your answers in narrative form. Imagine that this information is being communicated to a colleague who will be seeing the patient after hours.

Exercise 1 — Monique

Monique is a 28-year-old woman with schizophrenia. Her boyfriend has recently left her and staff in the supported accommodation home in which she lives report that she is tearful, distraught and withdrawn. They wonder if she is going to kill herself. The staff phone you and your task is to complete the risk documentation on the triage form. Refer to the template in Figure 9.1. The completed form appears in Appendix 3.

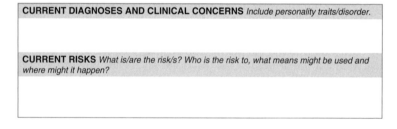

CURRENT DIAGNOSES AND CLINICAL CONCERNS *Include personality traits/disorder.*

CURRENT RISKS *What is/are the risk/s? Who is the risk to, what means might be used and where might it happen?*

Figure 9.1 Risk assessment and management template

Comment on the completed form

For Monique, she will need to be seen relatively urgently for a more complete assessment. The staff in the supported accommodation are anxious and part of the task of the assessment will be to manage this anxiety. Hopefully, she will already have a risk management plan which will make the process easier. This is how the risk may be documented in a triage form written by a duty worker receiving the call from the supported accommodation home. See Appendix 1 for an example of a triage form, including a place for documenting risk.

Exercise 2 — Phoebe

Phoebe is an 83-year-old woman with a major depressive illness characterised by delusions that her body is rotting, suicidal intent and psychomotor retardation. She has not eaten for 3 days. You see her in the ED.

Use the risk assessment template in Figure 9.1. The completed form appears in Appendix 3.

Comment on the completed form

Phoebe is at high risk. Documenting the risk in this way will facilitate admission to a hospital bed if there are resource limitations. Documenting the level of risk creates a requirement for monitoring to be set up at defined intervals of time. See page 26.

Exercise 3 — Colin

Colin is a 37-year-old man who has just moved from another city. You are asked to see him in the ED. He was brought in by the police after a report of a disturbance in the main shopping street where he was shaking his fist angrily at all and sundry and chanting. He is staring at you intently and says to you: 'There's nothing wrong with me'. There is a smell of cannabis in the room.

Use the risk assessment template in Figure 9.1. The completed form appears in Appendix 3.

Comment on the completed form

For Colin, the risk assessment starts immediately with your interpretation of his intent stare. His opening statement, 'There's nothing wrong with me', is likely to be made aggressively. Is this statement made because he is frightened or angry or both? His stare and the tone of his voice are important factors which will help in the identification of the potential risk and in the determination of its severity. Commenting on the lack of knowledge of whether a weapon exists or not is important for the continuing assessment. The answer has not commented on the smell of cannabis. Is he currently intoxicated? Is cannabis use a risk factor for violence — possibly not unless accompanied by psychosis. Does he have a psychotic illness related to substance abuse or is his psychosis possibly schizophrenia? There are a lot of unknowns in this example which will be common in an acute presentation.

Exercise 4 — Rebecca

Rebecca is a 26-year-old woman with borderline personality disorder (BPD). She phones you at 4.30 p.m. on a Friday saying that she has had an argument with her boyfriend and is going to self-harm. You know that she has razor blades in her bag. She asks you what you are going to do about it.

Use the risk assessment template in Figure 9.1. The completed form appears in Appendix 3.

Comment on the completed form

In this example, it is likely that, because Rebecca is already known to staff, she will have a risk management plan and possibly a crisis plan in place. This should give guidance about how to respond in this type of situation, which will be a recurring pattern of behaviour for Rebecca. Her somewhat aggressive approach may cause staff to become defensive or aggressive in turn, which may increase the risk. The other problem is that many patients who self-harm do not see the behaviour as risky. In fact self-harming may be seen as an effective solution to control overwhelming emotions. In these situations, there is often a large discrepancy between the assessment of level of risk as seen by the patient, their family and clinicians.

Discussion of exercises 1–4

You have been given limited information in the examples in these exercises. Nonetheless, being able to document the risk will assist in developing an immediate plan to deal with the crisis and, once the patient has stabilised somewhat, consideration can be given as to whether a more complete assessment needs to be undertaken. This is developed further in Chapter 11.

The following exercises extend the risk assessment and include the assessment of the static and dynamic risk factors. You are now being given more information and will need to practise documenting the risk factors. To help you, a list of risk factors for suicide accompanies the example of Monique and factors for violence accompany the example of Colin. The development of the risk factors is described in Part 3.

Exercise 5 — Monique (continued)

Refer to exercise 1 (page 76) for Monique's story.

BOX 9.3 RISK SCREENING

Practice points
- Documenting the risk allows for a degree of objectivity which reduces anxiety.
- Predicting when it may happen is difficult.
- If uncertain about whether to complete a full risk assessment, do it. If the risk is minor, the time spent will be small.
- An index of suspicion should be taken into all interviews to prompt for risk as patients will often not disclose risk issues spontaneously.

Monique's illness is characterised by both positive and negative symptoms. She continues to have auditory hallucinations which comment on her actions and occasionally put her down. Sometimes her voices tell her to hurt herself. Her self-care has deteriorated over the last few years, she has lost some of her outgoing vivaciousness and she has fewer friends. She continues to smoke cannabis from time to time. Six years ago, she became pregnant and had a termination. One year later, she became pregnant again and the baby was adopted out. She now uses a depot injection for contraception.

In her childhood, she says that she was happy and describes no major problems. She cannot remember too much about her childhood. She did not do well at school and left at the age of 16 with no qualifications. Monique's father has a diagnosis of schizophrenia. Her mother is well and she visits Monique about once a fortnight.

In her history, Monique has made three serious suicide attempts. The first attempt was 5 years ago and the last one 18 months ago. On each occasion, she was suffering a relapse of her schizophrenia and took overdoses of her medication.

Monique was in a relationship with another resident at the hostel.

Two weeks ago that relationship broke down after the boyfriend had a relapse and became violent. Since then, Monique has been frequently tearful and has withdrawn. Staff at the hostel have always felt that Monique is vulnerable to abuse by others but now say that they have a gut feeling that she is suicidal.

From the information given, document the current risk. Identify static and dynamic risk factors which will help you in your assessment of the risk of suicide. Include the protective factors. Use the risk factors for suicide in Table 9.1 to help you. Are there any patterns?

Table 9.1 Suicide risk factors

Risk factors for suicide

Static factors
- Male gender. Ratio approx 4:1. Age groups 15–24 and over 60.
- Previous attempt. If previously attempted, 10–20% will succeed.
- A history of neglect or sexual abuse.
- Substance use disorder.
- Family history of suicide.
- A history of self-harm.
- History of mental disorder.

Nature of the risk
- Well formulated or poorly developed plan?
- What means have been considered?

Illness (dynamic) factors
- Current suicidal ideation, communication and intent. Feelings of desperation, abandonment, hopelessness, rage, self-hatred or anxiety.
- Co-morbid depression. The more severe the illness, the greater the risk.
- Current alcohol use.
- Other psychiatric illness with affective component.
- Physical illness.
- Current diagnosis of personality disorder, especially borderline and antisocial personality disorders.
- Impaired rational thinking: especially schizophrenia and psychosis.

Situational factors
- Isolation, loneliness.
- Recent suicide of friend, family member or public figure.
- Recent loss — bereavement, divorce or job.
- Recent experience of adversity or stressful event.
- In youth, an identifiable stressful event precedes 70% of suicides.

Protective factors
- Has the patient previously sought help?
- Therapeutic alliance? Family support?
- Concerns about the effect of a suicide on others.
- Awareness of early warning signs.

Table 9.1 Suicide risk factors—cont'd

Risk factors for suicide
Systemic factors
• Do others think there is a problem?
Early warning signs and triggers
• What has indicated or triggered events in the past? Can the patient recognise their triggers?
• Does the patient have good or poor insight into his/her illness?
Relapse indicators
• Does the patient or his/her carers recognise indicators of relapse?
• Will the patient accept treatment voluntarily?

As you do this exercise, imagine you are discussing your thinking with Monique.

Use the template in Figure 9.2, over the page. The completed risk assessment and management form appears in Appendix 3.

Comment on the completed form

The box focussing on past episodes of risk yields very important information which would be a major focus for any clinician seeing Monique out of hours. A clinician seeing Monique for the first time would use this information carefully in their assessment of the level of risk.

The answers given for the static risk factors above ('What in this person's history …') have been documented in the form of a running list. Although they may be correct, they are difficult to read and if you are the clinician on call at night being asked to see Monique, it would be easy to skip over the static risk factors and focus more on the current mental state, situational and protective factors which have been documented in a narrative form.

BOX 9.4 CLINICAL TIP

When documenting risk, think about your colleague who will be seeing your patient after hours. Whilst trying to be succinct, it is sometimes easier to read when put in a narrative form rather than a running list, or list of dot points, or a series of tick boxes.

CURRENT DIAGNOSES AND CLINICAL CONCERNS Include personality traits/disorder.

CURRENT RISKS What is/are the risk/s? Who is the risk to, what means might be used and where might it happen?

PREVIOUS EPISODES OF THE RISK(S) Where did it happen, to whom and when? What was the context — illness, situational factors, substance use, not taking medications? Document each episode in as much detail as possible. Identify recurring patterns (risk scenarios) from this information.

WHAT IN THIS PERSON'S HISTORY CONTRIBUTES TO INCREASING RISK? For example, history of substance use, conduct disorder, impulsivity etc. Use the validated scales from your training manual.

WHAT MENTAL STATE FACTORS INCREASE THESE RISKS? For example, hallucinations, delusions, feelings of rejection, depression etc.

Identify early warning signs and triggers of these factors. Who notices the changes first?

WHAT EXTERNAL, ENVIRONMENTAL OR SITUATIONAL FACTORS AFFECT THE RISK? For example, substance use, living conditions, relationship problems, not taking medication etc.

WHAT SKILLS OR RESOURCES ARE THE PROTECTIVE FACTORS? For example, insight into illness, supportive family, stable accommodation, compliance with medication etc

Figure 9.2 Risk assessment and management template

Exercise 6 — Colin (continued)

Refer to exercise 3 (page 77) for Colin's story.

In ED, Colin allows you to take a history. There is a significant family history of abuse, mental health issues and substance misuse. For the last 10 years Colin has been smoking five joints of cannabis per day and tends to drink between 10 and 20 cans of beer per week. He says that approximately 6 months ago, he felt that his flatmate became more interested in his girlfriend and wondered if the flatmate was putting cameras in the ceiling to watch him making love to her. Initially he thought that this was a ridiculous idea but he became sufficiently concerned over a period of time to start checking around his room for hidden cameras and tape recorders. Shortly after this, Colin developed an unshakable idea — the newsreader on the television was giving him special messages.

These thoughts went on for some time and became more problematical for him. His girlfriend thought he was going crazy and left. In the end, Colin decided to leave his flat and moved to your town to start afresh. He has no family support in your town and finds himself wandering the streets where he recites prayers to try and distract himself from thinking that people are talking about him. Approximately 1 month ago, Colin noticed that when he smoked more cannabis, the 'paranoid' ideas became stronger and he wondered if the cannabis was the problem. He has used speed (methamphetamine) occasionally. He decided to stop the cannabis and, over the last few weeks, the paranoia has settled slightly, but it has certainly not gone away. Colin has found himself wondering if people on the streets are talking about him and has also wondered if his new flat mate is watching him. Colin has past convictions for assault; when he was 19 years old and again at 21 and 24. He tells you that he has learned to control himself since that time and wouldn't hurt anybody now. These assaults occurred in the context of brawls, which he got into when he was drunk. He says he normally wouldn't hurt a fly.

Colin says that he is getting increasingly angry about what is going on. Despite your best efforts to persuade him to take medication, Colin feels that he can manage this on his own using willpower and prayer. He thanks you for your help and says that he will be all right.

From the information given, document the current risk, identify static and dynamic risk factors which will help you in your assessment of the risk of violence. Include the protective factors. Use the risk factors for violence in Table 9.2 to help you. Are there any patterns? As you do this exercise, imagine you are discussing your thinking with Colin.

Use the template in Figure 9.2. The completed risk assessment and management form appears in Appendix 3.

Table 9.2 Violence risk factors

Risk factors for violence

Static factors

- Male gender and younger age of first violent incident.
- Past history of violence. Consider the degree of violence and the frequency.
- Substance use. Is this historical and/or is it continuing today?
- Childhood maladjustments and behavioural problems and childhood abuse.

Nature of the risk

- Risk to whom, type of weapon? Well formulated or poorly developed plans?
- Predatory or affective type of violence?

Illness (dynamic) factors

- Psychosis — is the patient threatened, frightened and are normal controls overridden?
- Does the patient feel persecuted?
- Is the patient having command hallucinations?
- Changing symptoms. A tendency to act on symptoms.
- Impulsivity. Lack of Insight.
- Violent thoughts being expressed? Morbid jealousy?
- Threatening or fearful behaviour.
- Current diagnosis of personality disorder — especially psychopathy but include antisocial personality disorder.
- Self-report of thoughts of violence.

Situational factors

- Current substance use.
- Unstable accommodation. Unemployed. Current stressors.
- Poor compliance with medication. Poor therapeutic alliance.
- Access to weapons.

Protective factors

- What has worked previously to prevent violence?
- Good therapeutic alliance.
- Family support?
- Concern about harming others. Awareness of triggers.

Table 9.2 Violence risk factors—cont'd

Risk factors for violence
Systemic factors
• Do carers think there is a problem?
• Is the situation at home deteriorating?
• Is the treatment plan feasible?
Early warning signs and triggers
• What has helped in the past?
• Does the patient have good or poor insight into his/her illness?
• Can the patient recognise their triggers?
Relapse indicators
• Does the patient or their carers recognise indicators of relapse?
• Will the patient accept treatment voluntarily?

Comment on the completed form

It is tempting to say that Colin has a drug-induced psychosis but this is not known yet. Mental health clinicians have a poor record of using this diagnosis in a pejorative way, causing both stigma to patients and also poor treatment. Documenting the signs and symptoms of illness is often more useful when completing risk documentation as colleagues will look for these after hours. In the section of the form allocated for early warning signs, reference has been made to Colin moving towns. Good practice will allow for risk assessments and plans to be readily available to clinicians in different areas of the country. Early warning signs are often subtle indicators that appear before full-blown symptoms of illness have emerged. Note that the reciting of prayers is both protective for Colin and an indication that he is ill. If you are seeing Colin after hours the prompt that he may check for recording devices can be useful as it is a non-verbal sign and does not require good rapport.

Discussion of documentation of risk assessment

Completing these exercises will give you some familiarity with the process of doing a risk assessment. Using the risk tool makes it easier for other clinicians, the patient and their family to make use of the information. However, for clinicians doing routine assessments, it can be time consuming to complete the documentation in this format. In some circumstances it may be sufficient to document the risk in a narrative form as a paragraph with the simple heading, 'Risk Assessment'. Two examples appear below.

Example 1: Alternative risk assessment record

Alan reports difficulties with chronic thoughts of suicide and depressive symptoms, however he has a number of plans for his future that appear realistic and many of these are in relation to preventing relapse. He did not describe a sense of hopelessness and his risk to self was assessed as currently being low. Should Alan relapse back into alcohol use and his previous lifestyle, his risk to self would elevate to at least moderate.

Alan does not report recently increased irritability, although he has a past history of aggression towards others and impulsivity. His risk to others was currently assessed as low–moderate, and this risk would also increase should he relapse into substance use.

Example 2: Alternative risk assessment record

While Richard experiences fleeting suicidal thoughts, he has no current intent and the actual thought of dying scares him. He has never made any self-harm attempts in the past. I feel his current risk to himself is low but there is the potential that if his depression and anxiety worsens, his drug use continues, or if he is faced with serious psychosocial stress, given his impaired ability to problem solve and his tendency to catastrophise (see glossary), this risk may increase. It therefore needs to be monitored. There is no risk of harm by him to anyone else and no concerns about his current ability to care for himself.

Despite his mental illness and drug dependence, Richard has recently managed to complete a degree in engineering, start a job and get promoted after 6 months. He has the insight to realise the impact his opiate use is having on his ability to function and on his mental state, and is motivated to achieve abstinence.

Comment

In both of these examples, which were taken directly from patients' notes and de-identified, the current risks have been identified and consideration has been given to the static and dynamic and protective factors. Both of these examples have commented on the level of risk. Unfortunately it is not clear what low risk or low–moderate risk means from these examples. In the first example, the critical factor of relapse into substance abuse has been identified. The second example recommended that the risk be monitored although there was no timeframe mentioned. Also, in the second example multiple risk factors have been

BOX 9.5 RISK ASSESSMENT

Practice points

- Structured clinical judgment (SCJ) combines clinical information and actuarial information known to be of relevance.
- SCJ allows for ease of review by others and is reproducible.
- Good risk assessment lays the foundation for good risk management.
- Good risk assessment should make it easier for the patient and family to share the risk and to participate in risk management.
- Good risk assessment should identify repetition of internal and situational factors, which are highly significant.[6]
- Signature risk signs and critical risk factors should be identified.
- 'Risk scenarios' — situations or states of mind where the risk is more likely to occur — should be identified.
- When uncertain, consider taking advice from colleagues, seeking supervision, getting a second opinion or discussing the case in the multidisciplinary team (MDT).
- Discussing risk openly with your patient does not increase the risk.
- When documenting risk, using a narrative style is easier for colleagues to read.[7]
- Imminence of risk is assessed at each meeting with the patient and is guided by the risk management and treatment plan.

identified with no particular critical factors noted. In neither example was the management of the risk documented. It is hoped that this was included in the management section of these patients' documentation!

The problem with documenting risk in this way is that it may be difficult to find it in the body of the notes later.

If need be, both of these examples could be adapted and put into the risk tool quite easily if it was thought the patient may present after-hours or in a crisis. Some clinicians might say that risk should always be documented separately and placed in the file in a place which is easily seen. This is discussed further in Chapter 11.

Notes

1 Murphy D 2002 Risk assessment as collective clinical judgment. *Criminal Behaviour and Mental Health*, 12:169–78.

2 Gutheil TG, Schetky D 1998 A date with death: management of time-based and contingent suicidal intent. *American Journal of Psychiatry*, November. 155:1502–57.

3 Maden A 2007 *Treating Violence: a Guide to Risk Management in Mental Health.* Oxford University Press, Oxford.

4 Veale D, Freeston M, Krebs G, Heyman I, Salkovskis P 2009 Risk assessment and management in obsessive-compulsive disorder. *Advances in Psychiatric Treatment*, 15:332–43.

5 Williams J 1988 A database method for assessing and reducing human error to improve operational performance. In: Hagen W (ed.) ILEEE *Fourth Conference on Human Factors and Power Plants*, Institute for Electrical and Electronic Engineers, New York: 200–31.

6 Winestock M 1996 Risk assessment. 'A word to the wise'? *Advances in Psychiatric Treatment*, 2:3–9.

7 Higgins N, Watts D, Bindman J, Slade M, Thornicroft G 2005 Assessing violence risk in general adult psychiatry. *Psychiatric Bulletin*, 29:131–3, 3–9.

10 The decision-making process

> Since we are unable to predict the future, the best we can do is to assess the patient and present reasonable treatment alternatives.[1]

In clinical practice, difficult decisions are made every day. It is never a situation where the decision is between one pathway that has no risks and another that has multiple risks. No treatment decision will be risk free. As a clinician, the need to weigh the risk associated with one intervention against the risk of other interventions is nearly always present. The intervention chosen is the one which has the potential for the best outcome for the patient despite the risk, or the intervention seems clinically to carry the least risk.

For example, look at the treatment decisions to be made in the following scenarios.

- If an inpatient is granted home leave, what is the likelihood of him not returning and what might be the consequence? Should he remain in hospital?
- A woman with schizophrenia has not been seen for 4 days. Should the police be asked to look for her?
- An actively suicidal patient does not wish to be admitted to hospital and his family want him treated in the least restrictive environment. Should he be admitted involuntarily?

There is a myth that the decision-making process will determine the outcome.

Clinicians cannot control or predict all the people and circumstances the patient will meet after they have left the office. Tragic outcomes do occur even after good and robust decision-making. Clinicians can only be responsible and expect to be held accountable for the decision-making process and its implementation, *not* the outcome. Most decisions can be defended if there is a record of having considered the alternatives. If a clinician has conferred with a colleague, and can demonstrate this in the notes, the likelihood of the decision being defensible is even greater. Clinicians should not be held accountable for the contributing factors over which they have no control.

Heuristics

The process of decision-making using insights from the field of cognitive psychology has useful implications for risk assessment and management. Heuristics as a method of decision-making were introduced briefly in Chapter 2. Heuristics are 'cognitive shortcuts that allow decisions to be reached in conditions of uncertainty',[2] or 'rules that guide cognitive processing to help make judgments'.[3]

- Heuristics reduce the time, resources and cognitive effort required to make a decision.[4]
- They are a feature of mature clinical thinking[5] and are useful particularly when time and information are limited.
- Heuristics are more likely to be used when there are situations of high complexity or uncertainty,[6] when there is a high cognitive load or a high density of decision-making,[7] and when time for individual decisions is short.[8]

These are all situations when decisions about risk management may be made. However, reliance on heuristics leads to cognitive bias and 'severe and systematic errors'[9] and these have now been termed 'cognitive errors'[10] or 'heuristic biases'. The opposite process of using heuristics is one of rational-deductive decision-making in which all necessary evidence for and against any potential course of action is carefully examined and weighed. This assumes no bias on the part of the decision-maker and also assumes optimal time and resources.[11] Errors are more likely to be made using heuristics than when rational-deductive decision-making is used.

Heuristics can be seen as being closely allied to the concept of intuitive decision-making based on 'what feels right' or so-called 'gut feelings'. The differences between intuition and reason in decision-making can be outlined as shown in Table 10.1.[12]

Table 10.1 Intuition and reason in decision-making

Intuition	Reason
Fast	Slow
Effortless	Effortful
May be emotionally charged	Emotionally neutral
Opaque	Transparent

For many risk decisions made in everyday life, such as whether to cross the road or not, heuristics are used. We have neuropsychological systems responsible for such automatic choices,[13] based on habits derived from practice or from cognitive associations that have been learned over time. As is readily apparent, the capacity to make choices quickly has substantial adaptive value, but if the situation has changed subtly or if there are variables that have not been factored in, heuristic biases may creep in. There is a need to check the cognitions that are used for heuristics on a regular basis otherwise errors will creep in because of personal bias. To complicate matters, the use of heuristics is characteristic of doctors with good clinical acumen[14] so the best practice that is recommended is that, as far as possible, heuristics should be used consciously with an awareness of their pitfalls.[15]

Examples of heuristic biases, or cognitive errors[16]

- 'What I have experienced is more likely.' For example, 'this patient is just like that man I treated last year who ended up killing his father so he must have a very high risk of violence'.
- 'What I can remember is more likely.' For example, 'we have had three patients abscond in the past 6 months; this man seems likely to abscond if we let him out without an escort'.
- 'What I can easily imagine is more likely.' For example, dramatic episodes such as a heinous crime by a psychiatric patient can have a disproportionate influence on future decisions.
- 'What I want is more likely.' For example, mental health clinicians do not want bad outcomes so they may underestimate the likelihood of a patient being violent.
- 'What I expect is more likely.' For example, 'he seemed very pleasant, so I didn't ask him about plans to harm other people'.

Other forms of heuristic biases include:[17]

- Hindsight bias. Ignoring 'gut feelings' and not exploring them sufficiently.
- Ignoring relevant factors such as base rates data and contextual factors.
- A tendency to reinterpret difficult situations to resolve *cognitive dissonance* (see glossary). For example, a diagnosis may be modified so that the dissonance between 'a public commitment to care for needy people' and 'an inability to care for this needy person because of resource constraints' can be resolved.

The best process for decision-making is likely to be one where heuristics are utilised in conjunction with rational-deductive decision-making.

It is not always going to be possible to use a slow, deductive process but, equally, clinicians are not going to be able to take cognitive shortcuts until the slower rational-deductive process has been utilised on many occasions. Once this has occurred, heuristics (i.e. the cognitive short-cuts) can be utilised more frequently, as long as possible biases are considered. When this occurs, heuristics are likely to function maximally. Utilising the risk thermostat (Figure 6.1, page 45) when making decisions about risk may facilitate increased consciousness of heuristics.

For a more complete list of heuristics and their strengths and weaknesses see Crumlish and Kelly (2009).[18] For a more detailed exploration of heuristic biases (cognitive errors) when making risk decisions see Carroll (2009).[19]

The risk/benefit analysis (rational-deductive decision-making)

A lot of the time, clinicians use heuristics and weigh up whether the intervention is going to be administered at the right time, whether the patient is ready for the intervention, whether they can manage the insight gained.

For junior practitioners or when the possibility of heuristic bias is present, the slower process of rational decision-making can be a very useful option. In this method risks and benefits are carefully considered. The risk/benefit analysis is an iterative process about deciding which treatment option to take. It may occur during the assessment or during management and should be considered as a tool to be utilised whenever uncertainty exists. When the treatment option has been chosen and implemented, the outcome will be reviewed and further options considered in another risk/benefit analysis. This follows the thinking of Carson's (1996) 'Risk Path' in which a series of small 'steps' are taken.[20] The evaluation should consider the benefits and the opportunities presented by the situation as well as the risk. There will be situations where there will be high risk but also potentially better outcomes. There will also be situations where the obligation to protect society from a potentially violent person is in conflict with the patient's right to be treated in the least restrictive environment. These situations of cognitive dissonance need to be evaluated carefully.

There are several phrases that are commonly used to acknowledge that a risk has been considered.

- 'The benefits of taking this course of action outweigh the risks.'
- 'We need to take risk in the short term for long-term gain.'
- 'I weighed up the risk factors and made a clinical judgment.'

These are all examples where a risk/benefit analysis has occurred.

It is not uncommon for an individual clinician or a team to become hamstrung in their treatment because the risk issues seem insurmountable or the risk issues seem to take precedence. The risk/benefit analysis focuses on the opportunities involved when choosing treatment directions whilst taking risk issues into account. It is a useful tool to use when the options are unclear or if there is disagreement within the clinical team. This can be either in the acute situation or in circumstances when time is not paramount.

Utilising a risk/benefit analysis is an effective, straightforward and easily documented way of evaluating the treatment options involved. It is especially useful when clinicians are anxious about the consequences of the risk; for example, if one staff member says, 'we can't do this, it's too risky'. If a clinician on the team is risk-avoidant, using risk/benefit analyses as a team exercise can help immensely. It facilitates a more objective exploration of the situation.

In situations where there is risk or a certain amount of trial and error, or uncertainty, 'thinking out loud for the record'[21] can be useful. In the risk/benefit analysis the pros and cons, including known risks, advantages and disadvantages, are carefully documented. The reasons why a certain course of action is taken will then be clear. This will improve transparency should there be a poor outcome, as the decision-making process will have been clearly documented. If there is a claim for negligence in the future, having a documented risk/benefit analysis in the notes can be protective.

Whichever option is chosen, it will involve taking a risk of some kind. Once the treatment direction has been agreed, it is usual for some on-going risk still to be present. Clinicians, patients, families and managers need a process for living with this as nobody can live in a risk free environment. The risk/benefit analysis helps generate an awareness of the degree of on-going risk likely to be involved which can then be addressed in risk management. In some literature, this is referred to as risk mitigation; that is, mitigating the consequences of risk outcomes if they occur. For example, trying to reduce access to the means for committing suicide or reducing the frequency of drugs being dispensed are ways of mitigating risk.

Apart from the risk/benefit analysis being a step which facilitates risk management, it has several other useful spin-offs:

- it identifies in detail not just the risks but also the potential benefits which may occur even if a risky pathway is chosen
- competing treatment perspectives can be considered

- sometimes risks which had not been considered come to light when this process is used
- it facilitates group discussion of risk issues and can be a useful therapeutic tool to use with patients and their families
- it allows full documentation of uncertainty and how that is factored into the decision-making
- it can become a forum in which moral, ethical, legal and human rights issues are taken into account.

With reference to the last bullet point, in the majority of cases, clinical, ethical and legal concerns are aligned. However, the potential for a risk-management pitfall looms when different values in the same system of thought compete, such as when the obligation to protect society from an imminently violent mentally ill person competes with the right to treatment in the least restrictive setting.[22]

The risk/benefit analysis is also a tool to help minimise the number of *false-positives*. False-positives are those situations where the risk behaviour is predicted to occur when in fact it does not. False-positives are tolerated in mental health services to protect life. It is important to try and minimise *false-negatives* (missing those who do go on to display the risk behaviour) by utilising good risk assessment. Risk events such as violence or suicide are rare events even in mental health settings. Predicting if and when they may happen is a difficult task. It is important to err on the side of caution but at the same time not be overcautious and end up denying patients their freedom.

Below is a case example with a model for documenting a risk/benefit analysis. As will be seen, it occurs after the assessment has been completed and knowledge of patterns and risk factors will be available.

Case example

Caroline is a married woman with two adolescent children. She is in the midst of a severe depressive illness with substantial suicidal intent. This is her fourth episode of depression and each episode has been marked by suicidal intent. She has been admitted to hospital on two previous occasions for brief periods of time but does not want to go to hospital. Her husband is supportive but works in a very busy job. Her parents live locally and give all the support they can. Refer to Table 10.2.

The risk/benefit analysis process should help clinicians, the patient and their family decide how to proceed with care and treatment.

It is not a process of reducing risk but a process of deciding which risks to take in the context of trying to help the patient get better.

Table 10.2 Risk/benefit analysis example

Treatment options	Risk	Benefit
(Option 1) Admit to hospital	Caroline regresses. She suffers from increased stigma. She feels alienated from her family.	Suicidality is monitored closely. Staff feel less anxious. Depression can be treated more assertively.
(Option 2) Treat at home	Suicidality is monitored less closely. Family gets more worried. More difficult to treat assertively.	Caroline is happier when she is at home. She is able to continue caring for her children. She is treated in the least restrictive environment.

The decision taken may be one of higher risk but the potential for a better outcome is seen as important. Once the treatment option is chosen, it is important to remember that in many situations it does not need to be implemented straight away. There will often need to be some planning and preparation undertaken before the treatment gets under way.

Risk Management is not just about trying to reduce the level of risk; it also involves helping the patient get better. Clinicians will often mull over many of the following questions before adopting a treatment and risk management strategy. Many of these questions can be included in the discussion during the risk/benefit analysis.

- What happens if we do nothing? For example, we don't prescribe the new medication, we don't discharge the patient. Are the consequences of not taking the risk poor or detrimental to the patient?
- What happens if we take the risk and the outcome is poor? Can we manage that in advance?
- Can we reduce the level of risk without affecting the outcome of treatment?
- What happens if we take a conservative approach? In the short term the risk may be reduced but in the long term the outcome may be poorer.
- Even if we can't reduce the level of risk, is it still worth taking the risk? For example, if we get a better outcome.
- Can the risk be managed in this setting?
- What is the cost in terms of: resources, the patient, the therapist, the team, the company, financial?

- Does it increase the risk to others?
- Is this risk a priority?
- Do we need to manage the risk now or can we plan how to manage it in 'x' days?
- Is the acute management the same as the longer-term management?
- Does the risk management enhance the treatment of the patient?
- Is my anxiety about the patient affecting my decision-making?

When these questions arise in routine clinical practice, a risk/benefit analysis will often help clarify uncertainty.

BOX 10.1 RISK/BENEFIT ANALYSIS

Practice points
- The process of balancing risk and benefit must be carefully documented.
- At times it is necessary to take risks in order to achieve the desired outcomes even if the level of risk is high. The other outcome may be chronicity or deterioration of the illness.
- It may be necessary to take short-term risks for long-term gain.
- A risk/benefit analysis brings the risk firmly into the context of the patient's illness.
- A risk/benefit analysis allows for consideration of protective factors.
- A risk/benefit analysis allows for consideration of a balance between civil liberties and public protection.

Several exercises for risk/benefit analyses have been included below as it is an important tool, which is often under-utilised.

Exercise 1 — Colin (continued)

Refer to Chapter 9, exercise 3 (page 77) and exercise 6 (page 82) for Colin's story thus far.

At the end of the interview, Colin has declined to take any medication and is making it clear to you that he does not need any further treatment and he can sort all his problems out on his own. You feel that you have developed a reasonably good rapport with him and he has said that he will come back to see you in a few weeks to let you know how he is going. On the other hand, you are concerned about the possibility of him acting on his delusional preoccupations and wonder if he needs to

Table 10.3 Risk/benefit analysis for Colin

Management and treatment possibilities	Risk	Benefit
Admit to hospital involuntarily		
Arrange follow-up sooner than the few weeks that Colin has suggested		

be brought into hospital for treatment involuntarily. He says that he can control his anger and will not be violent.

Complete a risk/benefit analysis for Colin (Table 10.3). The completed risk/benefit analysis chart appears in Appendix 3.

Comment

In your service, there may be other management and treatment possibilities such as a day hospital or a crisis respite bed. To explore these, it is simply a question of adding another row or several rows to the risk/benefit analysis and completing these. This process may take place as a discussion with a colleague in the Emergency Department (ED). The important thing is to document the thinking process 'for the record'.

The example of Colin is a common clinical scenario and the risk/benefit analysis will often throw up the same risks and benefits. However, the treatment option chosen will be dependent on many other variables at the time. In the acute situation and when dealing with a patient who is unknown, it is often difficult identifying dynamic risk factors. Most clinicians would prefer to undertake a fuller risk assessment in this type of situation before moving on to the risk/benefit analysis but if Colin is keen to walk out, there may be some pressure. The clinical tip in Box 10. 2 may help although caution is advised as it relies to a large degree on inference on the part of the clinician.

Exercise 2 — Fred

Fred is a 45-year-old man suffering from chronic schizophrenia. He has unremitting positive symptoms. You want to try a course of clozapine instead of the monthly injection of Haldol™. There are some worries about compliance.

Fill in the risk/benefit chart in Table 10.4. The completed chart appears in Appendix 3.

BOX 10.2 CLINICAL TIP

- In the acute situation, checking for **insight**, **judgment** and **impulse control** will help when weighing up the risk.
  This is a difficult tip to work with as the items require a high degree of inference on the part of the clinician. However, when it is considered in more detail, these prompts remind the clinician to check for dynamic risk factors of importance which can change rapidly.

Table 10.4 Risk/benefit analysis for Fred

Management and treatment possibilities	Risk	Benefit
Continue with Haldol		
Start clozapine		

Comment

This is a very common scenario which most clinicians will recognise. The risks are relatively small but the process is the same. Becoming familiar with the process will make it easier to do in a crisis.

Exercise 3 — Jane

Jane is a 32-year-old married woman who is 12 weeks pregnant. This is her first pregnancy. She is currently in a medical ward where she was admitted over the weekend as she had concerns about her pregnancy. The doctors have asked you to assess her as they are concerned about her mental state. When you see her, she is in a single room and her husband and her parents are also present. She immediately tells you that there is nothing wrong with her and that she has never felt better. When you ask her the reason for this, she says that since the angels came to visit her, everything has been all right. She then expands on this and tells you that the room is so full of angels that she wonders how you have been able to get into the room. She then tells you that you are the best angel of them all as you have the biggest wings! Her husband tells you that she has been like this for 5 days but says that she has been slightly different for the last 2 weeks. Although there is no past history of anything like this, her mother tells you that Jane had a brief psychotic episode 8 years ago which did not require hospitalisation and settled within 2 weeks. None of the family nor Jane can remember if she needed medication on that occasion. On talking to her further, there are no other symptoms and signs of psychosis and she does not seem to be suffering from a mood disorder. She is slightly preoccupied with the various angels in the room but other than this, you can detect no other abnormalities on mental state examination. The medical staff have cleared her and say that she can be discharged from their ward.

Jane and her family are adamant that she is well enough to go home and Jane agrees to take medication if you feel that it is necessary although she also says that she would prefer not to take medication. As the interview progresses, you find yourself confused as to what the diagnosis may be and how best to manage this situation as you have not come across anything like this before.

Do a risk/benefit analysis for as many management and treatment options that you can think of. Use the same chart format as per Table 10.4. The completed chart appears in Appendix 3.

Exercise 4 — Roger

Roger is a 32-year-old architect who has worked extremely hard to obtain a senior position in a big firm in the city. He came from a well-to-do family but was sexually abused by an uncle for 2 years between the ages of 8–10. He had been in a stable relationship with his partner, Joanne, for 3 years but this broke down 9 months ago when she was unfaithful. Roger became depressed initially but this revealed underlying traits of borderline personality disorder (BPD). Roger has taken several major overdoses and has been admitted to hospital on each occasion. He is currently in the inpatient ward and has self-harmed on one occasion in the ward and taken one overdose whilst on day leave. Complete a risk/benefit analysis, considering whether Roger would be better off staying on the ward longer or if his treatment should continue in the community. Use the same chart format as per Table 10.4. His depression is currently well treated and in remission. The completed chart appears is in Appendix 3.

Comment

Risk/benefit analyses can be routinely used as an integral part of treatment with patients with traits of, or who have, BPD. The analyses can help to expose conflict within the treatment team and facilitate greater objectivity in treatment.

Exercise 5 — alcohol and drug example (Gillian)

Gillian is 28 years old and in a de facto relationship with Nathan. She is currently being treated with methadone substitution at a dose of 115 mg per day. She has 3 take-away doses per week. She has three children from previous relationships, all of whom are in care. It is likely that she suffers from BPD with several traits of antisocial personality disorder. This has never been confirmed as she refuses to attend for a psychiatric assessment.

Physically Gillian is well. She has previously been treated with methadone but on each occasion was involuntarily withdrawn from the program for diversion or use of illicit drugs. The decision to put her back on methadone again was not taken lightly but it was felt that, on balance, Gillian would be better off with it. Nathan has just been released from prison and within 2 months Gillian tells you that she is pregnant again. When she is 16 weeks pregnant, she diverts her methadone again and gives it to a friend who injects it. The friend dies from an overdose.

Complete a risk benefit analysis about whether to continue with methadone treatment. Use the same chart format used in the previous risk/benefit exercises. There are likely to be more than two treatment possibilities. The completed chart appears in Appendix 3.

Comment

Treatment options always generate risks and benefits. This is true for every branch of medicine. As well as considering the risks generated by the treatment option, clinicians will also be considering how to reduce the risks generated by the illness. This example was taken from a real situation. Initially there was a large amount of disagreement within the treatment team, but as the risk/benefit analysis was undertaken using a whiteboard (and hence everybody could see all viewpoints clearly), the disagreement, anger and anxiety resolved. The process of using the skills of all members of the multidisciplinary team was central to this. The patient was then invited in to participate in the process and a treatment option was chosen. The process then moved on to working out how to implement the treatment option.

Notes

1 Miller MC, Jacobs DG, Gutheil TG 1998 Talisman or taboo: the controversy of the suicide-prevention contract. *Harvard Rev Psychiatry*, 6:78–87.

2 Crumlish N, Kelly BD 2009 How Psychiatrists Think. *Advances in Psychiatric Treatment*, 15:72–9.

3 Goldbloom D 2003 *Psychiatric Clinical Skill*. Elsevier Australia, Sydney.

4 Croskerry P 2002 Achieving quality in clinical decision-making: cognitive strategies and detection of bias. *Academic Emergency Medicine*, 9:1184–204.

5 Groopman J 2007 *How Doctors Think*. Houghton Mifflin Harcourt International Publishers, Illinois.

6 Tversky A, Kahneman D 1974 Judgment under uncertainty: heuristics and biases. *Science*, 185:1124–131.

7 Croskerry P 2002 Achieving quality in clinical decision-making: cognitive strategies and detection of bias. *Academic Emergency Medicine*, 9:1184–1204.

8 Groopman, above, n 5.

9 Tversky & Kahneman, above, n 6.

10 Crumlish & Kelly, above, n 2.

11 Crumlish & Kelly, above, n 2.

12 Carroll A 2009 How to make good enough risk decisions. *Advances in Psychiatric Treatment*, 15:192–8.

13 Kahneman D 2003 A perspective on judgment and choice. Mapping bounded rationality. *American Psychologist*, 58:697–720.

14 Croskerry P 2002 Achieving quality in clinical decision-making: cognitive strategies and detection of bias. *Academic Emergency Medicine*, 9:1184–1204.

15 Groopman, above, n 5.

16 Carroll, above, n 12.

17 Carroll, above, n 12.

18 Crumlish & Kelly, above, n 2.

19 Carroll, above, n 12.

20 Carson D 1996 Developing models of risk to aid cooperation between law and psychiatry. *Criminal Behaviour and Mental Health*, 6:6–10.

21 Gutheil TG 1980 Paranoia and progress notes: a guide to forensically informed psychiatric record keeping. *Hospital and Community Psychiatry*, 31(7):479–82.

22 Miller CM, Tabakin R, Schimmel J 2000 Managing risk when risk is greatest. *Harvard Review of Psychiatry*, 8:154–9.

11 Risk assessment: focus on documentation

Keep the language simple.

This chapter builds on the previous chapters and begins to add a focus on the function of the risk behaviour. It is useful at this stage to focus again on aspects of documentation before revisiting the risk tool.

Documenting the risk

The importance of documenting risk cannot be understated. From a medico-legal perspective, 'if you didn't write it, it didn't happen'.[1] In situations where there is risk, a certain amount of trial and error, uncertainty and so forth, 'thinking out loud for the record'[2] is a useful reminder. Documenting the risk also provides a framework for thought. It has been difficult to develop any one process which successfully incorporates everything to do with risk management into the routine clinical file. There are, however, a few principles of risk management which cannot be ignored. The findings from international inquiries state consistently that the most common failings are those of poor documentation and poor communication.[3] There is a medico-legal requirement to document well and clinicians put themselves and their patients at substantial risk when this doesn't happen.

Risk documentation may vary from just a couple of lines in the notes in simple cases to several pages in more complicated cases; these outline all the static, dynamic and protective factors etc and how these all blend together. In the acute situation, it may well be impossible to adopt a carefully considered approach but in the majority of situations within a mental health setting, risk can be evaluated over a period of time and the process of documentation can be an equally considered process.

Documentation of risk should be concise but contain enough detail as to be useful to a clinician unfamiliar with the patient; for example, those seeing the patient out of hours. The documentation should be useful and not something which is put in the 'file and forget' basket. As the document will also be shared with the patient, language the patient can understand should be used (i.e. without psychiatric terminology).

Risk documentation should always include management of the risk and interventions for the dynamic risk factors.

Exactly where risk is documented in the notes will also vary from case to case, depending on the needs of the patient, the degree of risk and the acuity of the situation. How this is achieved seems to vary from one service to another but useful themes that emerge are:

- risk assessments, no matter how brief, are copied onto a risk form and put into a separate compartment in the file
- risk documentation is written on different coloured paper
- all risk documentation is copied to the mental health crisis team
- as more information becomes available, this should be added to the risk plan incrementally
- if risk issues are incorporated into the assessment, these are given headings and put in a box.

See Figure 11.1 for examples.

Where mental health services have moved to electronic health records (EHR), this process becomes much easier as risk documentation can automatically be incorporated into the relevant areas of the EHR. Subheading boxes within the risk plan can be completed directly from the assessment. Similarly, subheadings from the risk plan — especially identification of early warning signs and triggers — can be pasted directly into the treatment plan ensuring that the treatment plan covers the management of the risk factors. Updating of risk and treatment plans becomes much easier.

> **Risk**
> *'Mary had a very difficult upbringing characterised by ... and her threshold for relapsing into her depressive psychosis with its associated suicidality is currently low.'*

> **Risk issues**
> *'Jason says that he has not been violent previously. However, he sometimes yells out at his auditory hallucinations and this has provoked responses from members of the public who assume that he is shouting at them. He hinted that this has caused him difficulty in the past as people have assumed he is being abusive towards them and they have been threatening in return. As he is actively psychotic currently and his alcohol abuse is also poorly controlled, his management plan will need to take heed of this possible scenario.'*

Figure 11.1 Examples of how risk is documented

BOX 11.1 RISK DOCUMENTATION — THE RISK PLAN

Practice points: what a risk plan does

- It documents that risk has been considered and assessed.
- It puts the risk into the context of the current illness (mental state factors and patterns).
- It allows for consideration of situational factors (and patterns).
- It documents protective factors.
- It lays the foundation for risk management
- When combined with the treatment plan, dynamic risk factors and signs of relapse will also be managed.
- It does *not* usually state a definitive plan of action but makes recommendations. Treatment decisions in the acute situation are left to the clinician on the spot.
- Documenting the risk in a risk plan becomes a component of treatment for the underlying illness.

The next five exercises continue the process of getting used to assessing and documenting risk. Consideration of the function of the risk behaviour is now introduced. As described previously, adding this detail provides more contextual information, which helps in the development of treatment interventions. This is very important in illnesses such as borderline personality disorder (BPD) where the risk behaviours may have different meanings for different people but exploring the motivation for the behaviour can be of value in most illnesses.

The only part missing after these exercises will be the introduction of interventions for the risk factors, early warning signs and triggers. When necessary, use the list of risk factors in Tables 9.1 and 9.2 (pages 80–81 and 84–85). Remember, it is more useful for your colleagues if you write in a narrative form but don't get carried away by writing a thesis! The idea is to be brief and succinct. A test of the usefulness of your documentation is to show it to a colleague and ask them if it makes sense. As you get used to completing these examples, you will begin to notice that they also help you highlight areas where the treatment will need to focus. To an extent, documenting the risk in the form of a plan will direct some aspects of treatment.

Don't worry about whether you get the information in the correct box. As long as you get the information down on paper, your colleagues will be able to make use of it. You may also find that the same information is documented twice. Once again, it's better that it's down on paper than not at all.

Exercise 1 — Depression and post-traumatic stress disorder (PTSD)

David, 42 years old, has been seeing you and the consultant psychiatrist for 3 months for a depressive illness which has not responded well to a mixture of cognitive behaviour therapy (CBT) and antidepressants. Both you and the psychiatrist have felt that there is something missing from the history but despite gentle questioning, David has not told you anything more. During a routine case management session, he begins to tell you a story of being sexually abused by a male teacher when he was 14 years old during a school camp. This new information has been prompted by him reading an article in today's newspaper about a similar event. David becomes very tearful and angry and at one stage during the session; you wonder if he dissociates (see glossary). Towards the end of the session, David says that he knows where the teacher lives. At the end of the session, David is feeling very raw and you arrange to see him later on in the week and tell him that you will talk to the psychiatrist about this new information. Over the next few weeks, David develops flashbacks, poor sleep and greater anxiety. His depression is possibly worse and he is increasingly preoccupied with the idea of vengeance. He says that he would certainly not kill himself until justice has been served on the man who abused him. He is frightened by the intensity of his violent feelings. He has thought of the idea of attacking the teacher but has not taken these thoughts further. He says that remorse would overwhelm him.

David lives on his own and has few friends. He does not wish you to talk to his friends. He says that he has not been violent in the past and he does not drink or use drugs. He says that he does not want to kill himself but wonders how long he can endure this torment. He has made no plans to kill himself. From the information given, complete the risk documentation form for David. Figure 11.2 contains a risk documentation template. The completed form appears in Appendix 3.

Comment

This example is not uncommon in routine clinical practice. The risks are of both suicide and violence and the two are interlinked. What the clinicians have not done here is explore the risks in sufficient detail. They will need to ask the patient what means he might use for suicide or violence, whether he has planned it, and what might happen if he met the teacher on the street. They will need to consider impulsivity and consider what may tip him over into a violent or suicidal act. Are there any critical risk factors and signature risk signs which may be of

CURRENT DIAGNOSES AND CLINICAL CONCERNS Include personality traits/disorder.

CURRENT RISKS What is/are the risk/s? Who is the risk to, what means might be used and where might it happen?

PREVIOUS EPISODES OF THE RISK(S) Where did it happen, to whom and when? What was the context — illness, situational factors, substance use, not taking medications? Document each episode in as much detail as possible. Identify recurring patterns (risk scenarios) from this information.

WHAT ARE THE FUNCTIONS OF THE RISK BEHAVIOUR? For example, acting on delusions or hallucinations, self-harm reducing tension or distress; violence or threats being effective.

WHAT IN THIS PERSON'S HISTORY CONTRIBUTES TO INCREASING RISK? For example, substance use, conduct disorder, impulsivity, etc. Use the validated scales from your training manual.

WHAT MENTAL STATE FACTORS INCREASE THESE RISKS? For example, hallucinations, delusions, feelings of rejection, depression etc.

Identify early warning signs and triggers of these factors. Who notices the changes first?

WHAT EXTERNAL, ENVIRONMENTAL OR SITUATIONAL FACTORS AFFECT THE RISK? For example, substance use, living conditions, relationship problems, not taking medication etc.

WHAT SKILLS OR RESOURCES ARE THE PROTECTIVE FACTORS? For example, insight into illness, supportive family, stable accommodation, compliance with medication etc.	**WHO ELSE IS INVOLVED IN THE CARE AND TREATMENT OF THIS PATIENT?** Family, friends etc.

Have you put enough information in this form to help a colleague treat and care for this patient in an emergency?

Figure 11.2 Risk assessment and management template

importance? No early warning signs and triggers have been identified yet. The clinicians will need to meet to discuss this in some detail with David. However, it is important to start documenting the risk even if more details will be forthcoming later. The process of documenting the risk on a form often highlights areas of the history and current thinking that need clarification. The documentation on motivation for the risk behaviour carries vital information for a colleague caring for David after hours.

As can be imagined, the successful treatment of the underlying depression and PTSD will resolve the risks.

Example 2 — child and family example

Mike is an 8-year-old boy who has been referred to your child and family clinic because of secondary enuresis (bed wetting) and school phobia. This seemed to develop after the separation of his parents 6 months ago, although his brother and sister have coped well with the separation. He has been staying predominantly with his mother although he has each weekend with his father. His father's parents have also been helping out during this difficult time. When you see Mike on his own, he tells you in a somewhat shy, hesitant voice that everything is all right at home but he does wish that his parents would get back together again. He cannot account for his enuresis or school refusal and simply says that he does not like school anymore. Later on, you have a meeting with Mike and both his parents. His parents express appropriate concern but you begin to notice that Mike is much more hesitant and cautious in his interactions with his mother. At the end of the interview, you put your hand over Mike's shoulder to give him a friendly pat and he winces. Mike initially tells you that he fell over in the playground but after arranging a physical examination by his GP, the story begins to unfold that his mother has 'needed to contain him' at times when he puts up a fight about going to school.

From the information given, complete the risk documentation form for Mike. Refer to Figure 11.2 for a risk documentation template. The completed form and discussion appear in Appendix 3.

Exercise 3 — an example of using the model for exploring relapse prevention

Brian is a 45-year-old man with a diagnosis of schizoaffective disorder. His history is of several manic episodes complicated by auditory hallucinations, grandiose delusions and persecutory ideation. Not infrequently, the psychotic symptoms continue after the mood component has settled. The auditory hallucinations are variable in their content. Sometimes they tell him he is wonderful and can do anything he wants and at other times they have a paranoid flavour to them and tell him that he is being watched.

Brian has very little insight into his illness and prefers not to take his prophylactic medication all the time. He takes it more often than not though, as he says it helps him sleep. When manic, Brian is overactive, grandiose and disinhibited. The last time he was ill, he 'borrowed' a race horse from the local stables and rode it bareback to his home. Brian has not been violent previously but can be impulsive and at times verbally aggressive. He says that he doesn't really have an illness but his long suffering wife says that she can pick up the early signs of a relapse from his behaviour. She says that apart from the sleep disturbance, she 'knows' when he is getting ill.

From the information given, complete the risk documentation form for Brian. Refer to Figure 11.2 for a risk documentation template. The completed form and discussion appear in Appendix 3.

Exercise 4 — alcohol and drug example

Rachel is 34 years old and married to Jeremy. They have two children aged 8 and 4. Rachel has been alcohol dependent for nearly 6 years and also suffers from generalised anxiety disorder and occasional panic disorder. In her history, she was brought up in a loving, caring family who remain very supportive of her. When she was 19, Rachel was date raped but says that she has got over this. She has been treated in the local alcohol and drug service and currently takes naltrexone and paroxetine but there are substantial concerns about her compliance with these medications.

Four months ago, Rachel had a major relapse into alcohol use and, after smashing the family car and falling down the stairs, she voluntarily admitted herself to a residential program. For the first 6 weeks of the 8-week program she participated little but in the last 2 weeks, she began to participate and acknowledged that she no longer loved her husband and that the date rape caused her to avoid sex and also gave her nightmares. Since returning from her residential treatment, Rachel has again relapsed and says that she will not go back to residential treatment again. She says that she will be able to sort things out in her counselling. She has not told her husband about her feelings about the marriage. Her liver function tests are surprisingly normal. Although you have advised her not to drive, her husband tells you that she is still driving her children to school.

From the information given, complete the risk documentation form for Rachel. Refer to Figure 11.2 for a risk documentation template. The completed form and discussion appear in Appendix 3.

BOX 11.2 CLINICAL TIP

Alcohol is a major factor for both violence and suicide and other risks. Other substances, especially stimulants such as amphetamines, also create problems. It is current use which creates major difficulties at the time of assessment. Usually the difficulty is intoxication but a patient experiencing acute withdrawals can also have a lowered threshold for impulsive actions.

- A general rule of thumb if a patient is intoxicated at the time of assessment is to assume that a thorough mental state examination cannot be completed until the patient is no longer under the acute influence of the drug.
- Intoxication may well mean that the patient needs to be contained in a place of safety until sober.
- Policies and memoranda of understanding should be in place between mental health services, Emergency Departments (EDs) and police to manage this common occurrence.
- Clinicians should make a point of getting a collateral history from friends and family at these times.

Exercise 5 — opioid substitution example

Melanie is 35 years old and is a patient on your opioid substitution program and is prescribed methadone. She is hepatitis C positive but is otherwise well. She has a long-standing needle fixation and tends to inject her Sunday dose, which she picks up on Saturdays because her local pharmacy is closed on Sundays. The next nearest pharmacy, which is open on Sundays, is 25 km away. Melanie survives on a sickness benefit and says that she cannot get to the other pharmacy on Sundays. Melanie has diverted her weekday dose from time to time in order to inject. She is currently in a de facto relationship with Greg. He is on the waiting list for the opioid substitution program but the current wait is around 6 months. He has been assessed for the program and tells you that he is using morphine 30–60 mg every 2–3 days.

From the information given, complete the risk documentation form for Melanie. Refer to Figure 11.2 for a risk documentation template. The completed form and discussion appear in Appendix 3.

Notes

1 Gutheil TG 1980 Paranoia and progress notes: a guide to forensically informed psychiatric record keeping. *Hospital and Community Psychiatry*, 31(7):479–82.

2 Gutheil, above, n 1.

3 Maden A 1996 Risk assessment in psychiatry. *British Journal Hospital Medicine*, 56:78–82.

12 Risk management

> Psychiatric risks (chiefly violence to self or other) are manifestations of suffering, and addressing the suffering is the primary way psychiatrists and other mental health care workers should address risk.[1]

Risk management in a mental health setting is the task of minimising the likelihood of an adverse outcome whilst maintaining a focus on good treatment.

The quote below first appears at the beginning of the book, but it is useful to cite it again here as the message is very important.

> Much medical effort goes into managing the risks of complications of disease processes rather than managing the symptoms of the disease itself. Hypertension is the classic example, with no symptoms but plenty of treatments, all aiming to reduce the risk of complications such as strokes and myocardial infarctions. Psychiatry's misfortune has been to choose diseases where the complications … are homicide, suicide or reduced capacity for self-care and vulnerability.[2]

This problem becomes the nub of risk management within mental health. On the one hand clinicians try to treat the illness whilst at the same time managing the risk which is often a complication of the disease process rather than a symptom of the disease itself.

Given the examples that have been worked through in this book, it will be apparent by now that risk management is a combination of all the processes that have been described so far. The task now is to combine them into a whole and ensure that the effectiveness of the risk management can be evaluated.

Risk management on its own is meaningless. It is only when it is incorporated into the treatment of the patient's illness with a focus on recovery that it develops meaning. Before considering anything else, consider the illness. Sometimes in mental health there is no choice but to live with high risk whilst instituting appropriate treatment for the illness. This is no different to any branch of medicine. A pitfall in risk management for clinicians is instituting containment to reduce the risk which does not necessarily improve the outcome for the illness and which may also generate other risks.

EXAMPLE

A common example would be the risk-avoidant clinician with a very low threshold for admission to hospital who unwittingly creates dependence in his or her patients. The dependence created may lead to deterioration of the illness, possibly to chronicity and to further risk.

Trying to incorporate clinical management into risk management tends to lead to an approach in which the illness takes secondary importance. It is more effective to incorporate risk management into clinical management.

Risk management starts from the beginning of the first assessment and continues until the patient is discharged. It involves a series of decisions, some small and some large, made with the patient and often their family over the course of their path through mental health services.

> The clinician does not need to predict behaviour in the next 5 years or even 6 months, but only until the next outpatient appointment or home visit by the community psychiatric nurse.[3]

Imminence and level of risk is assessed during each meeting with the patient and is guided by the risk management plan. (For inpatient settings, this may be formally undertaken on a daily basis but in an outpatient setting, this should occur each time the patient is seen.)

As well as routine management of clinical risk, good risk management should also be able to cover the following situations:

- calculated risk-taking when the level of risk will remain high
- situations in which staff anxiety will remain high
- situations in which it may be contraindicated to reduce the level of risk
- situations in which the proposed management is counterintuitive.

EXAMPLE

The classical situation in which these bullet points arise is when a management plan for a patient with chronic suicidality is first implemented. The plan will often encourage a focus of the patient taking more responsibility for themself whilst continuing to get support from the mental health service. If the self-harming behaviour (e.g. cutting) has been reinforced by frequent long admissions to hospital or by extra phone calls, the shift of focus

---

may cause an escalation of self-harming behaviour in the short term. This should be anticipated and discussed with the patient who will be encouraged to utilise distress tolerance techniques that they will have been learning within their individual and/or group therapy. Nonetheless, there is a real risk of cutting becoming deeper, the patient feeling rejected, and the family being more concerned. The intuitive response is to not create more distress for the patient, which in the short term would help but in the long term would be negligent. Clinician anxiety during these times is often high. (See also the example of Sally, page 115.)

Risk management can be separated into two parts: management of the risk in the here and now and planning for the future. In practice, the two parts tend not to be divided as the management of the current situation should also be future oriented. A risk management plan can be used as a 'decision support tool'[4] both in the acute situation to facilitate immediate intervention as well as for implementing interventions over a longer period.

The tasks of risk management (after the assessment is complete)

1 Decide which treatment option to take and which risk(s) should be managed.
2 Managing risk factors in the context of illness.
3 Managing any other contextual matters.
4 Managing the potential consequences (risk mitigation).
5 Communicate the plan to the patient, other clinicians involved and others involved in the patient's care.
6 Document, document, document.
7 Implementation.
8 Review and evaluation.

1 Treatment options and risk

This will occur after the assessment and may involve the risk/benefit analysis (see Chapter 10).

2 Managing the risk factors (specific strategies)

To recap:

Likelihood = static risk factors + dynamic risk factors

Once the decision has been made to follow a particular course of action, and the risk/benefit analysis has been documented, the management of the risk factors can be considered. This is no different to routine clinical practice.

The management of both the static and the dynamic risk factors is one which is discussed amongst the treatment team, the patient and family. The focus of trying to reduce the likelihood of the event occurring will invariably focus more on the dynamic factors as the static factors will not change. There is no rank order for predictors. The only change which may occur with the static factors is the patient's adaptation to them. 'The value for the clinician is in the interaction of the factors.'[5]

How frequently the risk factors are reviewed will be dependent on the setting. In services in which levels of risk are used, there should be a schedule for formal reviews to be undertaken whilst other services will determine the frequency of reviews dependent on clinical judgment. In either case, the process will be the same: a review of the risk factors. In services in which standardised rating scales are used, there will be specific risk factors which are reviewed on a regular basis. In those services in which structured clinical judgment is used without standardised rating scales, those risk factors specific to the patient will have been identified and can be considered individually. Some clinicians use simple scales — present, partially present or absent — whilst others may wish to review the efficacy of the interventions.

This step is usually indistinguishable from good clinical management of the disease process. As well as treating and managing risk factors, assessment and interventions for the early warning signs (EWS), triggers and relapse indicators should be undertaken. The aim of looking forward is to anticipate repetition of the context.[6] This is the stage when the patterns which were identified as making the risk behaviour more likely are managed. *This step is the central task of risk management.*

EWS and triggers which may make the risk behaviour more likely are not the same as risk factors. EWS are often more subtle signs, such as irritability, loss of self-care, pre-occupation, etc. These will often be noticed by others before the patient notices them. Developing an awareness of precursors of the risk factors makes the likelihood of early intervention more possible. There will often be overlap between the risk factors, EWS and triggers. In practice it does not matter where they are documented as long as interventions are developed.

Identification of early warning signs (EWS)

Example 1

Chris is a patient with bipolar affective disorder. He usually presents with episodes of mania but has had two episodes of major depressive disorder. He enjoys the early stages of his manic episodes as he has more energy, feels invulnerable and has lots of creative ideas which he would like to incorporate into his business. Because these ideas have not been thought through, when he has implemented them, the business has often lost large amounts of money. Most of his admissions for mania have occurred several weeks into a relapse and have necessitated involuntary admission. His wife notices the early warning signs of a relapse long before Chris does. She notices that he does not sleep well, that he becomes sexually demanding and that he takes a greater interest in fitness than is usually the case for him.

Example 2
John is a patient with schizophrenia, paranoid type. During previous episodes of illness he has hit members of the public for no reason that was immediately apparent. His parents, with whom John lives, have noticed early warning signs of John relapsing into illness and also being more likely to become violent. He withdraws into his room, becomes less communicative and tends not to join them at mealtimes. He begins to pick arguments with his father.

Example 3 — clinical example
Sally is a 24-year-old woman with BPD. Over the last 3 years, she has made repeated superficial cuts to both her forearms at times of distress. Her family have been very concerned that these are attempts at suicide, and on 12 occasions she has had admissions to hospital. Sally has become very close with two of the nurses on the ward.

In recent weeks, as a result of a review of her treatment, education for Sally and her family, and the implementation of dialectical behaviour therapy (DBT), Sally has agreed to utilise some different techniques to try and change the pattern of behaviour. Even though Sally and her family realise that this will be difficult, and that she may actually find herself cutting more frequently for a period of time, she says that she won't. In fact, much to her distress over the next 3 weeks, she does cut herself more frequently and it is only when she is able to identify how much she misses the two nurses on the ward within her individual therapy, and with her family declining to take her to the ED after each episode, that the frequency of her cutting diminishes dramatically.

Summary of specific strategies
Consideration will need to be given to the threshold for and imminence of the risk behaviour occurring. The concepts of *signature risk signs* (page 20), *critical risk factors* (page 20) and *risk scenarios* (page 34) will help in this regard. For example, if an impulsive patient has a history of

being violent with little obvious provocation, violence may always be close by. For other patients, it may take immense provocation for them to become violent.

Sometimes it may be necessary to put short-term measures in place to reduce acute risk whilst waiting for the illness to settle.

A risk management plan will *always* complement and be a component of a fuller clinical treatment/management plan. The risk documentation should be placed in the patient's file in such a way that it is easily accessible for all clinicians and written in such a way so that the risk factors, early warning signs and relapse indicators can be cross-checked against the patient's mental state and external circumstances on the day that they are seen. Working with the patient and their family so that they all have copies of the risk and treatment plans makes this easier. This will also go a long way to increasing the likelihood of the management plan being feasible, the patient having better support and being less likely to be exposed to destabilising influences. These latter three factors rate highly in the Historical/Clinical/Risk Management 20-item (HCR 20) scale[7] risk management part of its scale as being of importance in preventing future episodes of violence.

Consideration should always be given to strengthening the protective factors. This is now being explored in one standardised rating scale.[8]

Note: The treatment plan as well as the risk management plan must include interventions for all the identified dynamic risk factors. The risk factors need to be contextualised where possible to the patient's illness and their own perspective on recovery.

3 Managing contextual factors

The physical context in which treatment is taking place, the time of day, clinician and team factors will all need to be considered. Management of these factors makes the management plan more feasible. It may be necessary to document how certain external contextual factors, such as lack of resources which are precluding optimal treatment, have been managed. (See the example.)

> **EXAMPLE**
>
> The optimal treatment for this patient would be 'a, b and c'. However, the resources currently available preclude this approach being taken and we have had to take an alternative approach — 'd'.

If this is documented in the notes, a clear message is being given that consideration of optimal treatment has been undertaken but because of resource implications, sub-optimal choices were necessary. This type of comment should be followed up by a letter to clinical leadership and management to alert them to the problem of insufficient resources.

4 Managing the potential consequences (risk mitigation)

After the treatment direction has been chosen, there will always be some risk left. Management of the potential consequences is primarily systemic and involves discussing the likelihood of the event occurring with the patient and family. It involves discussing the risk within the multidisciplinary team (MDT) and, if necessary, discussion with the wider management team. It will also involve the usual risk mitigation strategies such as limiting access to the means to complete the risk act; for example, limiting access to medication in the risk of suicidality etc.

Are the following questions able to be answered?

- Does the patient/family/company perceive the risk in the same way as the clinicians? Discrepancies in the perception of the risk by different people will cause substantial problems in the implementation of a risk management plan.
- How much responsibility can the patient or their family take at this time?
- Who is taking responsibility for the risk? Is it the clinician, the patient, the family? Is the responsibility shared? Does the family know the likelihood of death, suicide, assault, etc?
- Does the patient/family support the clinical approach? Patients and families are less accepting of risks over which they have little or no control, or where the consequences are dreaded. Patients and families are less likely to accept risks if there are no perceived benefits.
- Do senior clinicians support the approach? They will be the support if there is an adverse outcome. Do they even know what treatment approach is being followed? Do they need to know?
- Is there agreement from all on the level of risk?
- Will the management of the risk distract from, derail or complement the treatment of the illness?
- Has management of other risks been included; for example, media exposure?
- Consider: is a minor risk being managed because the major ones seem too hard to deal with?

5 Communicate to all concerned

This should be routine. For risk management plans, signatures of everybody who is involved in the treatment should be collected where possible. This is likely to include the patient, family, clinicians and possibly management. If this is not feasible, document who has been consulted in the development of the plan. Asking the patient to sign their plan is a therapeutic intervention, will improve rapport, ensure that the plan is feasible and also make it more likely that it has been written in plain English without 'psychobabble' (jargon) getting in the way. Signatories may also include chaplains, GP, medical wards, EDs and friends in more complicated plans.

Duty to warn and protect: a dilemma in communication

Occasionally a patient will threaten violence to a third party. The dilemma that a clinician finds themself in is: when can they breach patient–clinician confidentiality by informing the third party or legal authorities in order to protect them?

> The duty to warn and protect is a relatively new concept and is a departure from traditional psychiatric practice. This so-called duty is to a large degree defined by legislation and case law.[9]

The background case which generated the current focus on this issue was the Tarasoff case. In 1969, Prosenjit Poddar told his treating psychologist that he planned to kill his former girlfriend, Ms Tatiana Tarasoff. In response to this, the clinician provided both oral and written warnings to the campus police who interviewed Mr Poddar and subsequently released him. Mr Poddar later insinuated himself with Ms Tarasoff's family and then killed her. Her parents initiated a lawsuit. In the second court case, Tarasoff II, the court held that:

> … when a therapist determines, or pursuant to the standards of his profession should determine, that his patient presents a serious danger of violence to another, he incurs an obligation to use reasonable care to protect the intended victim against such danger. The discharge of this duty may require the therapist to take one or more various steps depending on the nature of the case. Thus, it may call for him to warn the intended victim or if it is likely, to appraise the victim of a danger, to notify the police, or take whatever steps are reasonably necessary under the circumstances.[10]

The onus on the mental health worker is to make him or herself aware of the current legal obligations with respect to duty to warn and protect. It is likely that this evolving area of law will continue to have a substantial impact on the care of the mentally ill.

There are some general guidelines that apply to most situations.

- A full risk assessment should be undertaken before any action is taken.
- The phrase 'if the release of that information is necessary to prevent or lessen a serious or imminent risk to others' should be considered as the litmus test for consideration of a breach of confidentiality.
- The clinical conundrum of differentiating between fantasy which needs to be discussed within the context of treatment and the reality of a threat of violence is a difficult area. It is likely that there is a continuum between fantasies of violence and direct threats.
- Laws about breaching confidentiality are slightly different in each country and, if uncertain, advice should be taken from a senior colleague or the legal services of the workplace.
- The person or group at risk needs to be identifiable.
- If usual clinical interventions such as admitting the patient to hospital cannot control the risk, it may be necessary to inform the third-party without the patient's consent in order to manage the risk. Only enough information to protect the third party should be disclosed. It would be rare that disclosure of psychiatric information would be required.
- Information may be passed on to an authority (e.g. the police) to protect the person at risk. If appropriate, the patient should be told that you are going to do this. If the patient's condition will worsen as a result, the patient should be told at a later time.
- This is a rare situation and the advice of senior colleagues should always be taken whenever possible.

For further reading see Gellerman (2005).[11]

6 Documentation of risk management

The level of risk is usually closely linked to acuity of illness. It is usually raised when a patient experiences deterioration of mental state or when situational factors re-occur. On the risk plan there should be spaces for documentation of risk factors, early warning signs and triggers along with recommendations for interventions should these occur in the acute situation. Although interventions may have been implemented to reduce the risk in the long term, crises can still occur. The risk management plan should include recommended interventions for these situations. The proposed interventions can only ever be recommendations. The final decision has to be left to the clinician on the spot because of the many variables which will need to be factored into each unique situation.

Many mental illnesses have an enduring nature and the associated risks will often be increased before florid signs and symptoms emerge. Frequently, the risks will be identified by family and friends. Incorporating this into a plan can be invaluable.

An intervention recommending admission to hospital — voluntarily or involuntarily — dependent on level of insight may be built into a risk management plan. Once it has been identified that the risks are more likely to occur with the onset of a relapse of illness, the issue of enforced compliance with medication will be raised. For those countries that have community treatment orders (CTOs) built into their mental health legislation, life has become easier as it is simpler to work with a seamless continuum between the community and hospital. However, there is a huge debate about the legal and ethical principles behind CTOs which may make their introduction in some countries less likely.

The debate about whether there should be a separate risk management plan or whether it should be incorporated into the treatment plan has not been resolved. If there is a separate risk management plan, at the very least interventions for the dynamic factors, early warning signs and triggers for relapse should be included in the patient's overall treatment plan as well.

Where possible, the patient should have a copy of their risk and treatment plans.

document, document, document

Consider the nearly fundamental truism: 'If it wasn't documented, it didn't happen'.[12]

Remember — the documentation in the clinical file is the judgment based on the information that was obtained by the clinician at the time. As long as the information available and the decision-making process was documented, the clinician should not be blamed for later events if the clinical decision-making was sound and well considered.

Example

In 1999 in Ballarat, Australia, a young woman committed suicide some months after discharge from hospital. She had a long history of substantial self-harming behaviour and a diagnosis of borderline personality disorder (BPD). The discharge planning from hospital had involved close consultation with the patient, her family and the wider system involved in her care. Everybody involved knew that there were substantial risks but it was also clear that prolonged inpatient hospitalisation was not improving matters. At the inquest, the coroner was able to review the extensive documentation and communication which occurred. His words were:

> … I am satisfied that the deceased received clinical, diagnostic, medicative, social and practical care and management at the highest professional level from these agencies.

The coroner went on to say:

> I wish to record the community's appreciations of the sustained support for the deceased offered by these agencies; and I record the following remarks made by the deceased's mother, in correspondence to the coroner's office:
>
> > 'I do not blame or criticise anyone for what has happened. It has been an extremely difficult situation. Grampians Psychiatric Services, Centacare and Ballarat Psychiatric Fellowship gave her everything and made a commitment to support her in every way possible. I only have praise for them.'[13]

Even when the outcome is adverse, clinicians do not need to be blamed.

7 Implement the plan in context of the treatment

Before implementing the plan, check that the future has been considered with reference to the past and present. Table 12.1 has a checklist to work through.

Table 12.1 Past, present and future checklist

Past	☑ Risk factors predisposing. Have these been considered? ☑ Previous episodes. Have patterns emerged?
Present	☑ Has the risk/benefit analysis been completed? ☑ Has a current assessment of level of risk been completed? ☑ Has current risk been reduced as far as possible? ☑ Have the risk mitigation strategies been implemented? ☑ Have risk factors for the future been identified? ☑ Is the illness being treated?
Future	☑ Have early warning signs (EWS) and triggers for future episodes been identified? ☑ Have interventions for EWS and triggers and relapse indicators been discussed? ☑ More commonly seen in forensic settings, has prediction of the likelihood of future episodes been undertaken?

8 Review and evaluate the effectiveness of the intervention

Set a date for the review. Make sure that this is communicated to everybody concerned. Preferably, review dates should be built into administrative processes.

BOX 12.1 RISK MANAGEMENT

Practice points
- A risk management plan should be placed in the patient's file in such a way that it is easily accessible for all clinicians.
- Managing the illness usually reduces risk.
- Imminence of risk is assessed at each meeting with the patient.
- Consider any contextual factors which may be of immediate relevance; for example, time of day, geographical situation, whether family are present, etc.
- Treatment of risk factors combined with assessment and intervention for the EWS, triggers and relapse indicators is the usual practice for reducing the likelihood of the risk behaviour occurring.
- A risk management plan will always complement and be a component of a fuller treatment/management plan.
- Consider the truism, 'If it wasn't documented, it didn't happen'.[14]
- The *treatment plan* should include interventions for all the identified dynamic risk factors.

The next two exercises in this section focus on the identification of interventions for the risk factors, early warning signs and triggers. The interventions are likely to be utilised in the treatment plan even if they are generated initially through the pathway of risk management. As described previously, the ability to 'cut and paste' makes the process of moving interventions from risk management plans to treatment plans easy. In the exercises, the plans have been partially completed. There is new information for both Colin and Monique and all that is required is for the early warning signs, triggers and interventions to be written in. Be creative with your answers and imagine that you are working alongside your patients whilst you are completing the exercises. The final part of the risk management form is a review of the efficacy of the interventions. Make sure you add a review date. This should be planned after determining how frequently the patient needs to be monitored.

Exercise 1 — Colin (continued)

You will remember Colin from Chapter 9 (exercises 3 and 6) and Chapter 10 (exercise 1).

The original example appears below, along with some new information.

Colin is a 37-year-old man who has just moved down from another city. You are asked to see him in the Emergency Department (ED). He was brought in by the police after a report of a disturbance in the main shopping street where he was shaking his fist angrily at all and sundry and chanting. He is staring at you intently and says to you, 'There's nothing wrong with me'. There is a smell of cannabis in the room.

In ED, Colin allows you to take a history. There is a significant family history of abuse, mental health issues and substance misuse. For the last 10 years Colin has been smoking five joints of cannabis per day and tends to drink between 10 and 20 cans of beer per week. He says that approximately 6 months ago, he felt that his flatmate became more interested in his girlfriend and wondered if the flatmate was putting cameras in the ceiling to watch him making love to her. Initially he thought that this was a ridiculous idea but he became sufficiently concerned over a period of time to start checking around his room for hidden cameras and tape recorders. Shortly after this, Colin developed an unshakable idea — the newsreader on the television was giving him special messages.

These thoughts went on for some time and became more problematical for him. His girlfriend thought he was going crazy and left. In the end, Colin decided to leave his flat and moved to your town to start afresh. He has no family support in your town and finds himself wandering the streets where he recites prayers to try and distract himself from thinking that people are talking about him. Approximately 1 month ago, Colin noticed that when he smoked more cannabis, the 'paranoid' ideas became stronger and he wondered if the cannabis was the problem. He has used speed (methamphetamine) occasionally. He decided to stop the cannabis and, over the last few weeks, the paranoia has settled slightly, but it has certainly not gone away. Colin has found himself wondering if people on the streets are talking about him and has also wondered if his new flat mate is watching him. Colin has past convictions for assault; when he was 19 years old and again at 21 and 24. He tells you that he has learned to control himself since that time and wouldn't hurt anybody now. These assaults occurred in the context of brawls, which he got into when he was drunk. He says he normally wouldn't hurt a fly.

Colin says that he is getting increasingly angry about what is going on. Despite your best efforts to persuade him to take medication, Colin feels that he can manage this on his own using willpower and prayer. He thanks you for your help and says that he will be all right.

At the end of the interview, Colin has declined to take any medication and is making it clear to you that he does not need any further treatment and he can sort all his problems out on his own. You feel that you have developed a reasonably good rapport with him and he has said that he will come back to see you in a few weeks to let you know how he is going. On the other hand, you are concerned about the possibility of him acting on his delusional preoccupations and wonder if he needs to be brought into hospital for treatment involuntarily. He says that he can control his anger and will not be violent.

New information

In fact, Colin returned 1 week later and said that he had changed his mind and would like to try the medication. He said that he was tired of hiding from people and questioning the way that people looked at him. Colin also said that he had come really close to hitting his new flatmate and didn't want to go to prison. He says that he was a bit of a brawler in the past aside from the 3 convictions and tended to use his fists as a way of resolving arguments. Colin was given some Risperidone and after 3 weeks felt much better.

Colin now says that he is back to his normal self and feels well enough to start smoking cannabis again! You express your concerns and start to talk to him about the nature of psychosis, the links with cannabis and begin to explore with him possible early warning signs of relapse and indicators that he may have relapsed. The trigger of cannabis use is one that you and Colin agree to discuss further.

Parts of the risk management plan (Figure 12.1) have been completed for you. Fill out some EWS, triggers and relapse indicators for the risk management plan. Use your clinical judgment to think of some interventions which may help. Add in a date for when you think the plan should be reviewed.

The completed plan appears in Appendix 3.

RISK ASSESSMENT AND MANAGEMENT FORM

		NAME OF PATIENT Place label here
DATE OF PLAN	25 June 2010	Surname: .... Given Name: Colin
REVIEW DATE (maximum — 6 months)		DOB: .... Patient ID number: ....

CURRENT DIAGNOSES AND CLINICAL CONCERNS Include personality traits/disorder.

Colin is suffering from a delusional disorder — paranoid type in which he feels that people are watching him. History of personality development is currently unknown.

CURRENT RISKS What is/are the risk/s? Who is the risk to, what means might be used and where might it happen?

Colin is at risk of being violent. The risk is most likely to be towards anybody whom he perceives as watching or persecuting him. He tends to use his fists rather than any weapon.

PREVIOUS EPISODES OF THE RISK(S) Where did it happen, to whom and when? What was the context — illness, situational factors, substance use, not taking medications? Document each episode in as much detail as possible. Identify recurring patterns (risk scenarios) from this information.

Colin was violent on three occasions in his late teens and early 20s. These all occurred when he was drunk and got into brawls in the pub. It's relevant to note that he was convicted on each occasion. In the past he had a low threshold for using his fists to resolve arguments.

Identify early warning signs and triggers of these factors.

WHAT ARE THE FUNCTIONS OF THE RISK BEHAVIOURS? For example, acting on delusions or hallucinations; self-harm reducing tension or distress, violence or threats being effective, etc.	**WHAT INTERVENTIONS HELP ADDRESS THESE FACTORS? WHAT SKILLS ARE BEING DEVELOPED TO DO THIS?** For example, reality orientation, self-soothing, cognitive skills, DBT skills, etc.
It is likely that Colin would only become violent if he felt that he needed to protect himself from perceived persecution by others. Violence in the absence of psychosis is unlikely unless he is drunk and gets into an argument although this has become less likely as he gets older.	

WHAT IN THIS PERSON'S HISTORY CONTRIBUTES TO INCREASING RISK?
For example, substance use, conduct disorder, impulsivity etc. Use the validated scales from your training manual.

Colin has had a low threshold for violence in the past, especially in the context of being drunk. He continues to use drugs, including alcohol. The last conviction was 13 years ago, however, and he is currently saying he doesn't want to go to prison.

Figure 12.1 Risk management plan for Colin (exercise 1)

WHAT MENTAL STATE FACTORS INCREASE THESE RISKS? For example, hallucinations, delusions, feelings of rejection, depression etc.	WHAT INTERVENTIONS HELP ADDRESS THESE FACTORS? For example, compliance with medication, reduced stress, etc.
Colin is most likely to be violent when he is suffering paranoid delusions or ideas of reference: he has felt that people are monitoring him with cameras and at times speaking to him from the television. If he is angry, this is probably a risk factor. *Identify early warning signs and triggers of these factors. Who notices the changes first?*	
WHAT EXTERNAL, ENVIRONMENTAL OR SITUATIONAL FACTORS AFFECT THE RISK? For example, substance use, living conditions, relationship problems, not taking medication etc.	WHAT INTERVENTIONS HELP ADDRESS THESE FACTORS? For example, respite, reducing drug use, phoning a friend.
Colin smoked cannabis until recently. If he restarts, this is likely to increase the risk. He also recently changed his accommodation and is not fully settled yet. He has recently started taking medication but if he stops this, the risk of violence will be increased.	
WHAT SKILLS OR RESOURCES ARE THE PROTECTIVE FACTORS? For example, insight into illness, supportive family, stable accommodation, compliance with medication etc.	WHO ELSE IS INVOLVED IN THE CARE AND TREATMENT OF THIS PATIENT? Family, friends etc.
Colin has some insight that cannabis abuse is problematical. He has recently stopped his cannabis use. He has not been violent since he was 24 and really wants to stay out of prison.	
Have you put enough information in this form to help a colleague treat and care for this patient in an emergency?	

Figure 12.1, cont'd

Exercise 2 — Monique (continued)

You will remember Monique from Chapter 9 (exercises 1 and 5). The original example appears below, along with some new information.

Monique is a 28-year-old woman with schizophrenia. Her boyfriend has recently left her and staff in the supported accommodation home in which she lives report that she is tearful, distraught and withdrawn. They wonder if she is going to kill herself.

Monique's illness is characterised by both positive and negative symptoms. She continues to have auditory hallucinations which comment on her actions and occasionally put her down. Sometimes her voices tell her to hurt herself. Her self-care has deteriorated over the last few years, she has lost some of her outgoing vivaciousness and she has fewer friends. She continues to smoke cannabis from time to time. Six years ago, she became pregnant and had a termination. One year later, she became pregnant again and the baby was adopted out. She now uses a depot injection for contraception.

In her childhood, she says that she was happy and describes no major problems. She cannot remember too much about her childhood. She did not do well at school and left at the age of 16 with no qualifications. Monique's father has a diagnosis of schizophrenia. Her mother is well and she visits Monique about once a fortnight.

In her history, Monique has made three serious suicide attempts. The first attempt was 5 years ago and the last one 18 months ago. On each occasion, she was suffering a relapse of her schizophrenia and took overdoses of her medication.

Monique was in a relationship with another resident at the hostel.

Two weeks ago that relationship broke down after the boyfriend had a relapse and became violent. Since then, Monique has been frequently tearful and has withdrawn. Staff at the hostel have always felt that Monique is vulnerable to abuse by others but now say that they have a gut feeling that she is suicidal.

New information

Unfortunately, over the next 3 weeks, Monique has a relapse of her schizophrenia with a worsening of her positive symptoms and increasing difficulty not acting on the voices which are now telling her to kill herself. She is increasingly withdrawn, uncommunicative and preoccupied with her psychotic experiences. Her self-care worsens and she is admitted to your inpatient unit for restabilisation and review of treatment. Over the next 3 weeks, Monique slowly settles and feels ready to return to her supportive accommodation. She is now also on an antidepressant as well as her antipsychotic medications.

Parts of the risk management plan (Figure 12.2) have been completed for you. Fill out some EWS, triggers and relapse indicators for the risk management plan. Use your clinical judgment to think of some interventions which may help. Add in a date for when you think the plan should be reviewed.

Comment

The immediate precipitants for Monique's current difficulties were the breakdown of the relationship with her boyfriend. The documentation in the risk management plan has not identified the importance of giving Monique some assistance and support to help her come to terms with the end of this relationship. Without this, it is likely that the risk of suicide will remain for some time. This is perhaps an example of the focus on risk overriding the need to help the patient manage the real problem, which in this case is the distressing end of a relationship.

The completed plan appears in Appendix 3.

RISK ASSESSMENT AND MANAGEMENT FORM

		NAME OF PATIENT	Place label here
DATE OF PLAN	25 May 2010	Surname: .... Given name: Monique	
REVIEW DATE (maximum — 6 months)		DOB: .... Patient ID number:	

CURRENT DIAGNOSES AND CLINICAL CONCERNS Include personality traits/disorder.

Monique suffers from schizophrenia with both negative and positive symptoms. She recently broke up with her boyfriend which has distressed her. She continues to smoke marijuana.

CURRENT RISKS What is/are the risk/s? Who is the risk to, what means might be used and where might it happen?

Monique has risks of relapse of her schizophrenia, suicide when her schizophrenia is uncontrolled and also after major life events.

PREVIOUS EPISODES OF THE RISK(S) Where did it happen, to whom and when? What was the context – illness, situational factors, substance use, not taking medications? Document each episode in as much detail as possible. Identify recurring patterns (risk scenarios) from this information.

When Monique becomes ill, her 'voices' often tell her to kill herself. She has made 3 serious attempts on her life by taking overdoses. The first occurred 5 years ago and the most recent 18 months ago.
Identify early warning signs and triggers of these factors.
Triggers for each overdose have been a relapse of her illness. Early warning signs are poor self-care, preoccupation with voices and upsetting events.

WHAT ARE THE FUNCTIONS OF THE RISK BEHAVIOURS? For example, acting on delusions or hallucinations; self-harm reducing tension or distress, violence or threats being effective, etc.	WHAT INTERVENTIONS HELP ADDRESS THESE FACTORS? WHAT SKILLS ARE BEING DEVELOPED TO DO THIS? For example, reality orientation, self-soothing, cognitive skills, DBT skills, etc.
Monique's capacity to ignore the 'voices' becomes less as her mental state deteriorates. She tends to act on the voices to stop them tormenting her and also because she tends to believe them when they say she must die.	

WHAT IN THIS PERSON'S HISTORY CONTRIBUTES TO INCREASING RISK?
For example, substance use, conduct disorder, impulsivity etc. Use the validated scales from your training manual.

Her chronic cannabis use makes it more difficult to control her schizophrenia.

Figure 12.2 Risk management plan for Monique (exercise 2)

WHAT MENTAL STATE FACTORS INCREASE THESE RISKS? For example, hallucinations, delusions, feelings of rejection, depression etc.	WHAT INTERVENTIONS HELP ADDRESS THESE FACTORS? For example, compliance with medication, reduced stress, etc
Monique is more vulnerable at times of major stress. Her hallucinations become more intense and frequent and her capacity to resist them is less. Monique is more at risk of suicide when her symptoms are more intense	
Identify early warning signs and triggers of these factors. Who notices the changes first?	
WHAT EXTERNAL, ENVIRONMENTAL OR SITUATIONAL FACTORS AFFECT THE RISK? For example, substance use, living conditions, relationship problems, not taking medication etc.	**WHAT INTERVENTIONS HELP ADDRESS THESE FACTORS?** For example, respite, reducing drug use, phoning a friend.
Monique continues to smoke cannabis and says that it helped her cope with the voices. Monique is very vulnerable to rejection. The inpatient environment is a 'safe' place for Monique. She tends to be at low risk when on the ward. Having access to more than 3 days medication is a temptation for Monique to take an overdose.	
WHAT SKILLS OR RESOURCES ARE THE PROTECTIVE FACTORS? For example, insight into illness, supportive family, stable accommodation, compliance with medication etc.	**WHO ELSE IS INVOLVED IN THE CARE AND TREATMENT OF THIS PATIENT?** Family, friends etc.
Monique's mother is supportive. The support staff are clearly concerned about Monique.	*Monique has the involvement of the community mental health team including her case manager, psychiatrist and psychologist. The staff at the supported accommodation house all like Monique and her mother is involved by visiting Monique weekly.*
SIGN & PRINT NAME & DESIGNATION	Date Time

Have you put enough information in this form to help a colleague treat and care for this patient in an emergency?

Figure 12.2, cont'd

Notes

1 Undrill G 2007 The risks of risk assessment. *Advances in Psychiatric Treatment*, 13:291–7.

2 Maden A 2005 Violence risk assessment: the question is not whether but how. *Psychiatric Bulletin*, 29:121–2.

3 Maden A 1996 Risk assessment in psychiatry. *British Journal of Hospital Medicine*, 56, No2/3.

4 McNeil D, Gregory AL, Lam JN, Binder RL, Sullivan GR 2003 Utility of decision support tools for assessing acute risk of violence. *Journal Consult Clin Psychol*, 71:945–53.

5 Maden A 2007 *Treating Violence: a Guide to Risk Management in Mental Health.* Oxford University Press, Oxford.

6 Grounds A 1995 Risk assessment and management in clinical context. In: Crichton J (ed.) *Psychiatric Patient Violence: Risk and Response*, Duckworth, London, pp 43–59.

7 Webster CD, Douglas KF, Eaves D et al 1997 *HCR-20: Assessing risk of violence* (version 2). Mental Health Law and Policy Institute, Simon Fraser University, Vancouver.

8 Webster CD, Nicholls TL, Martin ML, Desmarais SL, Brink J 2006 Short-Term Assessment of Risk and Treatability (START): The case for a New Structured Professional Judgment Scheme. *Behavioural Science and the Law*, 24:747–66.

9 Chaimowitz GA, Glancy GD, Blackburn J 2000 The duty to warn and protect — impact on practice. *Canadian Journal of Psychiatry*, 45:899–904.

10 Applebaum PS, Gutheil TG 1991 In: *Clinical Handbook of Psychiatry and the Law*, (2nd edn). Williams and Wilkins, Baltimore.

11 Gellerman DM, Suddath R 2005 Violent fantasy, dangerousness, and the duty to warn and protect. *The Journal of the American of Psychiatry and the Law* 33:484–95.

12 Gutheil TG 1980 Paranoia and progress notes: a guide to forensically informed psychiatric record keeping. *Hospital and Community Psychiatry*, 31(7):479–82.

13 Case of AB (1999). Ballarat Coroners Court. 129/1999.

14 Gutheil, above, n 12.

PART 3

RISKS OF SUICIDE, SELF-HARM AND VIOLENCE

13 Risk of suicide

Although the risk of violence has seemed to generate more interest within mental health settings over the last few decades, the risk of suicide is one which general mental health clinicians are much more likely to have to deal with on a regular basis. The links between suicide and mental illness are much closer than those between violence and mental illness. It is a given that mental health clinicians should have a solid grounding in the assessment and management of suicide risk. Although there is no substitute for the experience gained from time spent assessing and managing suicidal patients, the assessment skills can be taught and there is a large body of knowledge available in this area.

Although suicide is a relatively rare event, it is a devastating event for those close to the person who died. The low base rate of suicide makes it difficult to predict such a tragedy. Suicide is generally, although not always, associated with mental illness and 'effective treatment can reduce or abolish the risk of suicide in those cases'.[1]

The risk of suicide is usually acute and short lived (days or weeks), with the patient becoming low risk after a vigorous treatment intervention. However, chronic suicidality does occur, especially in patients with illnesses such as borderline personality disorder (BPD), and this is discussed in the next chapter.

Assessment

The assessment of suicide risk is similar to the assessment of other risks and includes a need for:
- a good rapport with the patient
- sensitivity, but also a willingness to ask difficult questions in order to be able to deliver good treatment.

Many junior clinicians (and some senior) are reluctant to ask patients too many questions about their suicidal intent, usually out of a mistaken concern that they will upset the patient. It is vitally important to remember that there is *no* evidence that assessing suicidality increases the risk in any way whatsoever. In practice, the process of catharsis is often healing and will reduce the risk in some instances. Once sufficient rapport has been established, clinicians should not avoid asking questions in as much detail as is necessary to fully assess the risk.

Suicidality is a deeply personal experience, which in many instances is kept secret by the patient. It is associated with despair, desperation, loss of hope, alienation and guilt — all emotional states which are often not spontaneously offered in the clinical interview and have to be elicited by careful and specific questioning. Family members are often kept in the dark by the patient and may not be so useful in the clinical assessment as they are when exploring the risk of violence. However, family members should not be forgotten as they know the patient better than the clinician and will be able to say how the patient is not their usual self even if they cannot pinpoint what the problem is.

Assessment of suicide risk as an outpatient is essentially an exploration of the risk factors but, for an inpatient, there are a few added complications that need to be borne in mind. For inpatients, the assessment of risk should be repeated at clearly defined intervals. There should be agreement within the treatment team that as far as possible, the same clinician or clinicians should be responsible for reassessing the risk. For some inpatients, if the risk is assessed too frequently, the patient can become irritated with the process and may begin to withhold information. Finding the balance between sufficiently frequent assessments and not overdoing it can be difficult. Being mindful of times of increased risk, such as improving from a psychomotor retarded depression, shift changes, or at the time of discharge from hospital is important. It is also important to bear in mind that for some patients, the objective signs of improvement can in reality be an indication that the patient has attained some peace of mind by having finally decided how and when to complete the suicidal act. Once again, good and thorough assessment can help. Occasionally, staff on a ward may find a particular patient difficult and find themselves unwittingly creating the same sense of alienation that the patient experienced in their own home (malignant alienation[2,3]). This is highly dangerous and there should be processes set up to reduce the likelihood of this happening.

Relying on intuition or using the phrase 'I have a gut feeling that they are suicidal' is poor practice and should be avoided.

Further reading on assessment of suicide risk

New Zealand developed guidelines in May 2003 and these are available from: www.nzgg.org.nz.

- Click on 'Publications', then 'Mental Health'. These guidelines are comprehensive, easily read and have appendices for assessment of patients in distress, assessment of risk of suicide and risk factors for suicide. The guidelines are written for the New Zealand culture but are applicable to most other cultures. They can be easily used in the clinical environment. 'Appendix 2: assessment of risk of suicide' has a very useful summary of questions that can be asked.

Goldney's book, *Suicide Prevention* (Oxford University Press, 2008), is a recently published resource that is likely to become a major resource for any clinician learning about suicide. Chapter 8 explores assessment of suicidality in more detail than is possible here.

Risk factors for suicide

The risk factors for suicide can be divided into static and dynamic factors in the same way as for other risks. The difference for suicide is that the static factors are less useful in terms of giving some idea about the propensity for the risk behaviour than in the case of violence. However, the most important static factor is gender. Males commit suicide approximately four times more often than females. Suicide literally means 'killing of himself' and the reference to killing is a reminder of the aggression which is required to complete the act. Historically it was the older age group who were more likely to commit suicide, but in the last 3 decades youth between the ages of 15 and 24 have become an increasingly significant age group in suicide statistics. Although suicides in the family are of some importance, as are some developmental factors, the most important factors are the dynamic ones of mental illness and substance abuse. A consistent finding in psychological autopsies is that 80–90% of people who commit suicide had a mental disorder, particularly depression and often with co-morbid alcohol use or abuse.[4] The severity of the mental disorder is also linked to the likelihood of the suicidal act being successful. Any mental disorder which has a mood component to it will lead to an increased risk of suicide. This is especially the case for depression of course, but bipolar disorders and schizophrenia also rank highly.

Alcohol, which is a depressant drug, is of great relevance in suicide. Up to 40% of patients with alcohol dependence will attempt suicide and up to 7% will die by suicide.[5]

Co-morbid personality disorder increases the risk as do multiple psychiatric diagnoses as well as some physical illnesses, such as lupus, HIV/AIDS and cancer.

Interestingly, cannabis abuse does not seem to be associated with an increased risk of suicide.

Moving closer to the suicidal act, access to the means to commit the act will be of importance. It is insufficient to ask how the patient has thought of killing themselves. Clinicians need to ask what preparations the patient has made as well. For example, if a patient has thought of hanging themselves, the clinician needs to ask if a rope has been bought, if they have thought where they would do it, if they have put the rope over the beam, whether they tried putting their head through the noose, etc. Patients rarely offer this information spontaneously but the information is vital and the sharing of the information is often cathartic for the patient.

There is likely to be an experience of desperation, hopelessness, abandonment, rage, self-hatred or anxiety.[6,7] Desperation seems to be of greatest import in this list of emotions. A sense of being trapped and of there being no way out is often present when the suicidal intent is high.[8] If a patient describes feeling alienated from his friends, family or himself, the risk will be higher. There is some recent evidence that a suicide syndrome may exist in its own right separate to suicide being driven by a mental disorder.[9] This highlights the importance of the emotions of desperation, rage and so forth, which are not always present in depression, so the possibility of a suicide syndrome is a reminder to look for these when assessing for suicidality.

If a patient says that their family will be better off without them, the likelihood of an attempt being made is high and immediate intervention is required. An enquiry should be made at these times about the potential of harm to others; for example, a spouse or children in those patients who feel that their family would be better off without them.

If a friend or relative has recently killed themselves, the risk is also raised.

Although risk factors are important, they do not tell the whole story and can never do so, as patients who are successful with their suicide take some secrets to the grave with them. Nonetheless, trying to develop an understanding of the meaning or purpose of the suicidal intent will help with planning interventions.

Standardised rating scales have been developed to rate suicidal intent[10] but have not found widespread usage at this time.

Management of suicidal risk

The basic tenets of managing suicidal risk are no different to other risks and will not be repeated here other than to reinforce that comprehensive assessment, containment of the acutely suicidal patient until the crisis is over and vigorous treatment of psychiatric illness are central.

Some clinicians still use 'safety contracts' to manage the suicidal patient. These are agreements made with the patient who 'guarantees their safety' over a period of time. There is *no* evidence that these are of any benefit and current practice is that they should not be used either for acute or chronic suicidality.[11, 12, 13]

Within most clinicians' careers, they will have a patient who expresses suicidal intent but with a timeframe added. For example, 'I'll be dead by March 23' or 'I won't see this Christmas'. This is a difficult situation which requires an exploration of the meaning behind the statement as well as consideration of transference and counter-transference responses. Some patients may make a statement such as, 'If you don't admit me, I will kill myself'. The anxiety and counter-transference provoked can easily be raised to such an extreme that useful interventions become impossible. It is important to remember that these are communications from the patient that need to be explored and cannot be managed until their meaning becomes clear. The initial anxiety on the part of the clinician needs management in the usual way, as described in Chapter 6. In these situations, experience is invaluable and, if this is a new experience for a clinician, the support and advice of colleagues should be sought. Further reading on this topic can be found in Gutheil's article on the subject.[14]

The risk factors for suicide appear in Table 9.1, pages 80–81.

Notes

1 The Assessment and Management of People at Risk Of Suicide 2003 New Zealand Guidelines Group and Ministry of Health. Online. Available: www.nzgg.org.nz (accessed 19 Nov 2009).

2 Morgan HG 1979 *Death Wishes: The Understanding and Management of Deliberate Self-harm*. Wiley, Chichester.

3 Watts D, Morgan HG 1994 Malignant alienation. Dangers for patients who are hard to like. *British Journal of Psychiatry*, 164:11–15.

4 Goldney RD 2008 *Suicide Prevention*. Oxford University Press, Oxford.

5 Goldney, above, n 4.

6 Hendin H, Maltsberger JT, Szanto K 2007 The role of intense affective states in signalling a suicide crisis. *The Journal of Nervous and Mental Disease*, 195(5):363–8.

7 Hendin H, Maltsberger JT, Haas AP, Szanto K, Rabinowicz H 2004 Desperation and other affective states in suicidal patients. *Suicide and Life Threatening Behaviour*, 34(4):386–94.

8 Williams JMG, Crane C, Barnhofer T, Duggan D 2005 Psychology and suicidal behaviour: elaborating the entrapment model. In: K Hawton (ed.) *Prevention and Treatment of Suicidal Behaviour*. Oxford University Press, Oxford, pp 71–90.

9 Fairweather-Schmidt KA, Anstey KJ, Mackinnon AJ 2009 Is suicidality distinguishable from depression? Evidence from a community-based sample. *Australian and New Zealand Journal of Psychiatry*, 43:208–15.

10 Bouch J, Marshall JJ 2005 Suicide risk: structured professional judgment. *Advances in Psychiatric Treatment*, 11:84–91.

11 Rudd MD, Mandrusiak M, Joiner T 2007 The case against No-Suicide Contracts: the commitment to treatment statement as a practice alternative. *Journal of Clinical Psychology: In Session*, 62:243–51.

12 Bateman A, Fonagy P 2006 *Mentalization Based Treatment for Borderline Personality Disorder*. Oxford University Press, p 48.

13 Boyce P et al 2003 Summary of Australian and New Zealand clinical practice guidelines for the management of adult deliberate self-harm. *Australasian Psychiatry*, 11(2):150–5.

14 Gutheil TG, Schetky D 1998 A date with Death: Management of Time-Based and Contingent Suicidal Intent. *American Journal of Psychiatry*, 155:1502–7.

14 Managing chronic risk

Chronic risk as a term is used predominantly to refer to a risk of suicide which remains present in a patient in a sub-acute form but which can become acute from time to time. It is also used for patients with repeated self-harming behaviour which at times is difficult to differentiate from acute suicidal risk. This behaviour is frequently linked to the diagnosis of borderline personality disorder (BPD) but is also seen in other personality disorders, dysthymia and chronic depression. The focus of this chapter is to look at the risk as it relates to patients with BPD although some of the techniques can be utilised in patients with other diagnoses when the same psychodynamic features are present.

The first part of this chapter outlines the medico–legal and clinical reasons why calculated risks in patients with chronic risk can be taken. There is then a brief outline of the process of taking a calculated risk followed by some ideas on the content of a crisis plan for patients who frequently self-harm and, finally, some clinical tips. The treatment of patients with borderline personality disorder is a much larger subject than can be addressed in this book and interested clinicians should consider reading books such as:

- Bateman A, Fonagy P 2006 *Mentalization-based Treatment for Borderline Personality Disorder: a Practical Guide*. Oxford University Press, Oxford.
- Krawitz R et al 2004 Professionally indicated short-term risk-taking in the treatment of borderline personality disorder. *Australasian Psychiatry*, 12(1):11–22.
- Linehan MM 1993 *Cognitive Behavioural Treatment of Borderline Personality Disorder*. The Guilford Press, New York.

Professionally indicated short-term risk-taking

Before embarking on the development of a plan for managing chronic risk, it is timely to remember that a diagnosis of BPD should not be made lightly. It is likely that a patient will have been assessed and treated within a mental health service for some weeks or months before the diagnosis is made and detailed assessments and formulations will have been undertaken. The clinical picture needs to be clear before management approaches for chronic risk can be put in place.

The risks most frequently associated with the BPD diagnosis are self-damaging acts and suicide attempts. Between 70 and 75% of people with BPD have a history of at least one self-injurious act and estimates of suicide rates vary, but tend to be about 9%.[1] Given the high frequency of suicide attempts, death by suicide is a genuine risk. This risk has been reported to be of the same magnitude as that noted in patients with schizophrenia or bipolar affective disorder (BPAD).[2] This data high-lights the risk clinicians face when working with BPD. *Self-harm exists on a continuum with suicide for the patient with BPD*.[3] The behaviour is not necessarily seen as being risky by patients. It is often the clinician or family member who sees the danger. The dynamic which leads to either self-harming behaviour or attempted suicide is difficult to explain simply. Individuals with BPD can experience a sense of badness which can be overwhelming. Self-harm can be understood as a way of using a physical act to relieve unbearable emotional states. The similarities with entrapment, which is a risk factor for suicide, are clear. Subsequent to the event, the patient often feels relieved and experiences a greater sense of self-coherence. Suicide attempts often occur when the patient is temporarily unable to mentalise (see glossary). The patient often believes that one part of them will survive the suicide attempt and that an alien/bad part will be destroyed.[4] Suicidality can vary from zero lethality and intent to un-ambivalent intent.[5]

For these patients, the behaviour is adaptive until such time that other ways of expressing distress are learned. For patients with BPD, the behaviour is likely to persist over time. This has substantial relevance to the issue of hospitali-sation as it is unlikely to change the level of risk substantially. Paradoxically, hospitalisation can increase the risk.[6, 7]

There are two important factors to consider in deciding how active to be in response to a suicidal crisis:[8]

1 the short-term risk of suicide if staff *do not* actively intervene
2 the long-term risk of suicide and of a life not worth living, if staff *do* actively intervene.

The response to the patient in any given case requires a good knowledge of dynamic risk factors and of the functions of suicidal behaviour for the patient. These are more clearly identified in patients well known to the service. For patients less well known, treatment will be more conservative and active.

Certain responses may in the short term decrease the probability of suicide, but that response may actually increase the likelihood of future suicide.[9] When suicidal ideation and threats are enacted because of the consequences they bring — that is, they function to get others actively involved (e.g. get help, solve problems, obtain admission to hospital, etc) — clinicians need to be careful that their response does not inadvertently reinforce the high-risk suicide behaviours they are trying to stop. Conversely when the suicidal behaviour is elicited in response to a situation or stimulus event, rather than by the consequences it brings, the behaviour will not be reinforced by responding to it. The nature of BPD is that the risk is likely to persist over time.

With a chronically suicidal patient, staff can expect a number of repeated suicidal behaviours before that behaviour comes under control. However, 'it is ultimately essential that the behaviour comes under the patient's control and not that of staff or of the community'.[10] 'Chronic suicide behaviour can be seen as being a mode of adaptation to life, an extremely common state among individuals with BPD.'[11]

If the patient is assessed to be an acute risk for suicide, then clinicians are ethically and legally required to take a directive role in preventing the patient from actually committing suicide — management of the short-term crisis is needed until the self-destructive phase passes. In contrast, chronic suicidal states driven by abnormal personality functioning represent a seriously disturbed yet consistent mode of relating to others and the environment by engaging others into assuming responsibility for suicidal behaviour and thus avoiding appropriate levels of personal responsibility for behaviour. Interventions for chronic suicide should assist and teach the patient to again assume realistic self-responsibility. Otherwise, traditional paternalistic and directive interventions may actually reinforce the destructive interpersonal dynamics of the individual with BPD and provoke further suicidal behaviour. 'Reducing risk to people with personality disorder involves placing a high degree of choice and personal responsibility with the patient.'[12]

'For both clinical and ethical/legal reasons, it is important that clinicians recognise the distinction between acute and chronic suicidal states.'[13] This differentiation needs to be clearly assessed and documented. If a chronic suicidal state is affirmed, clinicians need to actively employ a treatment approach based on the interpersonal context and avoid the use of traditional management approaches (longer-term voluntary or involuntary hospitalisation). Involuntary hospitalisation should only be considered when the chronic suicidal state crosses the boundary into an acute suicidal state. 'With the patient's informed consent, informing family members that their relative is chronically suicidal allows them to have realistic expectations for therapeutic progress.'[14]

It is important not to treat acute and chronic suicidal behaviour in the same way. Whatever the roots of chronic suicidality, prolonged inpatient care is likely to perpetuate and worsen their difficulties as independent, autonomous functioning decreases and dependency intensifies.[15,16] However, there is a dilemma for clinicians:

> we understand that repeated hospitalisation is not therapeutic, and that the patient needs to take responsibility for self, but patients certainly do commit suicide and to some extensive degree we are morally responsible for our patients, especially when their judgment is disturbed.[17]

The common belief that the responsibility for keeping the suicidal patient alive rests with the psychiatrist/clinician does not help and increases cautionary, but counter–therapeutic, practice. Prolonged hospitalisation is also likely to create an environment where the patient is more likely to experience 'affect storms' (see glossary) and this increases the likelihood of further self-harm.

> Such cautionary practice can lead to a worsening downward spiral of regressive attempts to get patients to take responsibility for their lives. Giving responsibility back to the patient, even though the immediate suicide risk may increase for a time, is the best hope.[18]

The turning point in the treatment of a chronically suicidal personality is often when suicidal feelings begin to be communicated freely, help in resisting them is asked for and reliance on externally imposed controls is given up. Well-considered, calculated risks are not reckless, they are necessary. This area of work is demanding and, for many clinicians, anxiety provoking. The risk of burnout is real and countertransference problems (see glossary) can undermine the best efforts. The importance of supervision for both individual clinicians and teams is central to working with patients who present with problems of chronic risk.

When is taking a calculated risk appropriate?[19]

When the clinician reaches an informed, considered opinion that precautionary, close-monitored management is no longer beneficial and is likely to lead to long-term worsening of the patient's condition, the responsibility for personal safety should be given back to the patient.

This is not only ethically defensible but therapeutically necessary. Clinicians must consider, in making this decision, if depressive, psychotic or substance abuse features have been treated appropriately.

How to take a calculated risk

The following steps are guidelines and are necessary for legal protection of the clinician responsible and of the institution.

- Short- and long-term risks and benefits of treatment have been clinically considered and are documented. (See the section on risk/benefit analyses in Chapter 10.) A formal consultation with an experienced colleague documenting support for the treatment plan, acknowledging the hazards of prolonged hospitalisation and that taking calculated risks is in the patient's best interest, is essential. The risk/benefit analysis should be reviewed regularly.
- The patient is assessed for acute or chronic suicide behaviour and this is documented. By the time clinicians are considering a professionally indicated short-term risk-taking approach, the patient will have (usually) had a history of a standard approach to suicidality and self-harm that will have been counterproductive, with negative outcomes.[20]
- A reasonable community treatment plan is devised. This should be based on a therapeutic alliance and help the patient to maintain a sense of responsibility without being rejected or rescued. It should include guidelines for crisis clinicians, pathways to respite and hospitalisation and the patient's individualised crisis strategies. It should be reviewed regularly.
- The patient understands and agrees to the planned treatment, and understands that taking a calculated risk is an important step in the treatment. Documentation must include that the patient is mentally competent to consent. (Depressed mood and delusions do not necessarily impair a patient's competency to make a reasonable decision. The issue of competency is beyond the scope of this book. Advice should be taken for definitions of competency.)
- Family and close friends need to be fully informed about the treatment plan and the inherent risks and benefits. The risks and benefits of prolonged hospital care should also be explained. The family agreement should be obtained and documented.
- It is important to be able to respond to changed circumstances. Changes in the pattern of suicidality, mental state changes, acute stressors and so forth should lead to an urgent review.

'At some future time will a malpractice action be brought asserting that overly restrictive, regression–inviting management negligently promoted, not prevented, suicide?'[21]

> There is a paradox in working with potentially suicidal borderline patients. Clinicians require the courage to face the possibility of a patient's death without losing confidence in their ability or their profession. Patients recognise this courage and grow more confident in its presence. Conversely timidity teaches the patient that life is just as scary as they always thought it was and may heighten the risk of actual suicide.[22]

The consensus in the reviewed literature is that traditional suicide management approaches may be therapeutically counterproductive, even dangerous in the long term, for the chronic suicide behaviour common among patients with BPD.

Crisis plan

Patients with chronic suicidality frequently present with crises. Indeed, the crises are times when patients often learn more about themselves and practise some of the techniques which they may have been learning in treatments such as dialectical behaviour therapy (DBT) or mentalisation based therapy (MBT). Because of the frequency of crises, it is not unusual for these patients to have a separate crisis plan which is appended to the overall treatment plan.

Before a crisis plan can be implemented, it is necessary to have discussed the diagnosis with the patient and also to have developed a formulation which helps organise thinking for both the mental health team and the patient. A well-structured formulation and treatment plan is therapeutic and lays the foundation for an effective crisis and treatment plan.

The crisis plan should follow the routine processes for risk management. As usual, it is necessary to identify the dynamic mental state and situational factors which make the risk behaviours more likely to occur. Early warning signs, triggers and relapse indicators should be identified and interventions planned for each situation. The balance between the patient taking as much responsibility as they can for each crisis and the patient's request for treatment is managed by planning for as many situations as possible in advance, and through clinical intervention.

- List and number the usual crisis situations, early warning signs and triggers; that is, feeling like self-harming, actual self-harming.
- Detail, under each crisis, the client's own response; for example, using self-soothing, coping strategies.

- Detail the mental health service response to each crisis for when the client is unable to manage independently.

Crisis cards, as forms of advanced directives, are sometimes used in these situations.[23]

Crisis phone calls[24]

At the outset of treatment, a clear message needs to be given that telephone calls are not therapy and should not be used in this way by either the patient or the therapist. Crises do occur, however, and patients do need to be able to phone if there is an urgent problem which they cannot resolve on their own. Some patients find phone contact easier than face-to-face therapy. This will need to be addressed if the pattern of avoiding therapy sessions and increasing phone contact begins to emerge.

Do not contact the patient to reduce therapist anxiety unless discussed with at least one other team member.

Clinical tips at times of crisis[25]

The therapist needs to:

- make a systematic attempt to place some of the responsibility for the patient's actions back with the patient with an aim of re-establishing self-control
- make clear that the staff are able and willing to respond to the emergency
- remain calm — anxiety in the therapist reduces his ability to mentalise (see glossary)
- sensitively monitor counter-transference and other responses
- assess the immediacy of the threat and consider it in terms of previous acts of self-harm or suicide attempts
- be aware of the well-known risk factors for suicide (see Table 9.1, page 80–81)
- keep talking to the patient about the feeling and its immediate precipitants
- be clear about the patient's role whilst the suicide risk remains high
- following the episode, ensure a thorough review in a number of contexts, including individual therapy, group therapy and with the multidisciplinary team (MDT).

Example

Figure 14.1 provides an example of a completed risk plan. As has been described earlier, these plans should be written using easily understood language, with minimal use of jargon. Descriptions of behaviours and mental states, such as 'she struggles to like her mum', are much more useful than using phrases such as 'she cannot introject good objects'. For patients with BPD, this is especially important as the patient needs to 'own the plan' and be an active participant in it.

A woman, Rebecca, has BPD and self-harms, and has chronic suicidality. In the 'Current Risks' box, there is a description of the paradoxical nature of the self-harming behaviour:

> Rebecca usually says at the time of cutting herself she wants to die and for the pain to go. She feels comforted by the thought of death being a release and is clear that if she didn't have that thought, life would be intolerable.
>
> Shortly afterwards, she can usually recognise that she doesn't want to die.

It is useful to try and document this in the plan. It could have been put in the box looking at the function/motivation for the behaviour if an intervention had been considered for the paradox.

Note: For most patients, this would be sufficient to cover the management of risky situations. However for patients with BPD, it is often necessary to develop a crisis plan which outlines the responses of both the patient and the staff to the scenarios which are usually predictable.

This plan stretches out to three pages despite the prompts being removed, which is common with chronic risk as the details become important.

RISK ASSESSMENT AND MANAGEMENT FORM

		NAME OF PATIENT	Place label here
DATE OF PLAN	1/4/2010	Surname:	Given name:
EXPIRY DATE (maximum — 6 months)	1/7/2010		*Rebecca*

CURRENT DIAGNOSES AND CLINICAL CONCERNS

Rebecca has a diagnosis of borderline personality disorder which she agrees with. She has difficulties with regulating her emotions and she sometimes self-harms by cutting when they overwhelm her. She has a past history of bulimia nervosa but this has resolved. She binge drinks alcohol occasionally.

CURRENT RISKS

Rebecca's self-harm behaviour causes risk of serious self-injury or even death.
Although most of Rebecca's self-harming behaviour is to relieve unbearable emotional states, there is also a risk that she may die. Currently, Rebecca carries a razor blade in her bag for security and does not want this taken away. Rebecca usually says at the time of cutting herself she wants to die and for the pain to go. She feels comforted by the thought of death being a release and is clear that if she didn't have that thought, life would be intolerable. Shortly afterwards, she can usually recognise that she doesn't want to die.
Rebecca's self-harming behaviour is a chronic pattern of risk (a repetitive response to life's difficulties) and is present whether she is in hospital or at home.

Figure 14.1 A completed risk plan

PREVIOUS EPISODES OF THE RISK(S)

Rebecca has self-harmed since May 2004. These are usually cuts across her arms which occasionally require sutures. This year, she has cut herself on her arms on five occasions. She has cut herself on her legs on three occasions this year but says that she doesn't plan to do this again as it hurts too much.

Rebecca recognises that she self-harms usually in response to difficulties within her relationships, especially with her boyfriend, but also with her mother and some other friends. She feels rejected at these times and very alone. Rebecca usually cuts in the toilet and tends to tell her mother a few minutes later, although she also says that she feels ashamed that she has cut again.

Over the last 5 years, the frequency of cutting has stayed relatively stable.

Rebecca has not self-harmed in any other way.

WHAT ARE THE FUNCTIONS OF THE RISK BEHAVIOURS?	WHAT INTERVENTIONS HELP ADDRESS THESE FACTORS? WHAT SKILLS ARE BEING DEVELOPED TO DO THIS?
Rebecca finds that her chronic preoccupation with suicide and death is soothing.	*Rebecca is practising distress tolerance techniques in her dialectical behaviour therapy (DBT) program. She is also practising attending to her wounds herself rather than asking her mother for help.*
By being monitored closely, Rebecca has felt cared for each time she self-harms which has been reinforcing.	*Hospitalisation does not prevent this risk and actually increases it by the process of reinforcement.*

WHAT IN THIS PERSON'S HISTORY CONTRIBUTES TO INCREASING RISK?

Rebecca's mother was hospitalised for 6 months when Rebecca was 3. When she was 10, an abusive stepfather moved into the home until she was 15. Looking back, Rebecca feels that she was always more 'sensitive' than her friends.

WHAT MENTAL STATE FACTORS INCREASE THESE RISKS?	WHAT INTERVENTIONS HELP ADDRESS THESE FACTORS?
Whenever Rebecca feels abandoned or rejected, she is at risk of self-harm. She often feels highly anxious and agitated when on her own. Rebecca tends to impulsively self-harm in response to these experiences. She tends to self-harm as a way of releasing the intensity of her emotional state. She has a low threshold for self-harming.	*Rebecca is learning to implement the training from her DBT treatment. She has a checklist to work through if she recognises her early warning signs and there is an agreed process for advice if she phones in crisis.*
Identify early warning signs and triggers of these factors. Who notices the changes first?	*Changes in the pattern of self-harming behaviour should lead to a review of mental state and consideration of acute suicidality. Rebecca may choose brief hospitalisation at these times (see crisis and treatment plans).*
Rebecca finds it difficult to identify the early warning signs of abandonment or rejection. She knows that when she is with other people, she can misread their intentions.	

Figure 14.1, cont'd

WHAT EXTERNAL, ENVIRONMENTAL OR SITUATIONAL FACTORS AFFECT THE RISK?	WHAT INTERVENTIONS HELP ADDRESS THESE FACTORS?
Arguments, especially with her mother or boyfriend, often trigger her core beliefs of unworthiness, inadequacy, and un-lovability. When these are triggered she becomes overwhelmed by her emotions. Frustration, anger and despair are all mixed up together. Rebecca is more likely to self-harm when she has been drinking or using drugs.	Rebecca has grounding techniques which she finds useful. She also is learning to implement chain analyses to rewind the process which led to the argument. The same process is implemented if she phones in crisis. Interventions for binge drinking and drug use are currently being discussed with Rebecca.
WHAT SKILLS OR RESOURCES ARE THE PROTECTIVE FACTORS?	**WHO ELSE IS INVOLVED IN THE CARE AND TREATMENT OF THIS PATIENT?**
Rebecca accepts her diagnosis and is working hard within her DBT group to reduce her self-harming behaviours. She has also said that she would like to be able to wear short-sleeve tops in the summer and have plastic surgery on her arms if she is able to stop cutting for 12 months.	Rebecca's management plan supports her taking as much responsibility for her self-harming behaviour as possible. Rebecca's family and mental health staff have tended to consider her self-harming behaviour as suicidal behaviour in the past. The approach of not taking immediate responsibility for Rebecca when she is agitated or self-harming may cause a short-term increase in risky behaviour, as she attempts to engage others to help her. However, this approach will reduce self-harm over time, as she learns that she can manage it.

TEAMS AND CLINICIANS INVOLVED

Beth Roberts, Case manager. Dr Waites, Psychiatrist. Denise McPhail, DBT key worker. All work in South CMHT. 04 XXX XXX

THIS FORM MUST INCLUDE A FACE SHEET & TREATMENT PLAN

COMPULSORY COPY TO: CATT AND MENTAL HEALTH LINE

ALSO COPIED TO: ☐ Patient   ☐ Family/Whanau   ☐ GP
☐ ED ☐ Accommodation Provider   ☐ Other (specify)

PRINT NAME AND DESIGNATION	Date
	Time

Have you put enough information in this form to help a colleague treat and care for this patient in an emergency?

Figure 14.1, cont'd

Notes

1 Linehan MM 1993 *Cognitive Behavioural Treatment of Borderline Personality Disorder*. The Guilford Press, New York.

2 Stone MH 1993 Paradoxes in the Management of Suicidality in Borderline Patients. *American Journal of Psychotherapy*, 47(2):255–72.

3 Linehan MM 1986 Suicidal people: One population or two? *Annals of New York Academy of Science*, 487:16–33.

4 Bateman A, Fonagy P 2006 *Mentalization-based Treatment for Borderline Personality Disorder: a Practical Guide.* Oxford University Press, Oxford.

5 Krawitz R et al 2004 Professionally indicated short-term risk-taking in the treatment of borderline personality disorder. *Australasian Psychiatry,* 12(1):11–22.

6 Maltsberger JT 1994 Calculated risks in the treatment of intractably suicidal patients. *Psychiatry,* 57:199–212.

7 Paris J 2004 Is hospitalisation useful for suicidal patients with borderline personality disorder? *Journal of Personality Disorder,* 18(3):240–7.

8 Linehan, above, n 1.

9 Linehan, above, n 1.

10 Linehan, above, n 1.

11 Fine MA, Sansone RA 1990 Dilemmas in the management of suicidal behaviour in individuals with borderline personality disorder. *American Journal of Psychotherapy,* 44(2):160–71.

12 Crawford MJ, Price K, Rutter D, Moran P, Tyrer P, Bateman A, Fonagy P, Gibson S, Weaver T 2008 Dedicated community-based services for adults with personality disorder: Delphi study. *The British Journal of Psychiatry,* 193:342–3.

13 Fine and Sansone, above, n 11.

14 Fine and Sansone, above, n 11.

15 Maltsberger JT 1994 Calculated risks in the treatment of intractably suicidal patients. *Psychiatry,* 57:199–212.

16 Paris, above, n 7.

17 Maltsberger, above, n 15.

18 Maltsberger, above, n 15.

19 Maltsberger JT 1994 Calculated risk-taking in the treatment of suicidal patients: ethical and legal problems. *Death Studies,* 18:439–52.

20 Krawitz, above, n 5.

21 Maltsberger, above, n 19.

22 Stone, above, n 2.

23 Sutherby K, Szmukler GI, Halpern A, Alexander M, Thornicroft G, Johnson C, Wright S 1999 A study of 'crisis cards' in a community psychiatric service. *Acta Psychiatr Scand,* 100:56–61.

24 Adapted fromBateman A, Fonagy P 2004 *Psychotherapy for Borderline Personality Disorder.* Oxford Medical Publications, Oxford University Press, Oxford, Appendix 2.

25 Above, n 24.

15 Risk of violence

> The most effective response to the risks of dangerous behaviour in the mentally ill is not to return to policies of greater control and containment but to improve the care, support and treatment delivered to patients in the community.[1]

Violence is probably the most difficult risk for mental health clinicians to assess. Whereas suicide and self-harm are very closely aligned with mental illness, violence is not. Suicide and self-harm assessments are the bread and butter of a clinician's work. Whilst violence assessments are less common for a general mental health clinician, they are routine for clinicians working in forensic settings. To further complicate matters, the assessment of violence in a forensic setting usually occurs after the event and takes place in a relatively controlled environment. For a general clinician, assessments for violence occur in a setting which is more fluid and in which there may have been no previous violence: altogether a different world. However, research which has occurred predominantly in forensic settings has much to offer mainstream mental health workers.

The subject of the nature of violence is a textbook in its own right and cannot be covered here. Aggression and violence has been extensively written about over thousands of years, including religious tracts, novels and textbooks. This provides a hint of the important role it plays in matters relating to the human psyche. Violence is a complicated area for mental health clinicians and has been the subject of much research in recent years. Understanding the role that aggression plays in the development of violence is central to this topic.

Most violence is perpetrated by those who are *not* mentally ill. Some understanding of the pathways leading to violence in those who are not mentally ill is a prerequisite for the comprehension of violence when the presentation is complicated by mental illness. Within mental health, De Zulueta's book (1993), *From Pain to Violence: The Traumatic Roots of Destructiveness*[2] is an excellent introduction to the subject. She explores the origins of human aggression and violence, and its links with attachment and trauma. Violence and its association with risk is covered in detail in Maden's book (2007)[3] and should be consulted for a more intensive analysis of the brief introduction in this chapter.

Introduction

Physical aggression peaks at perhaps around the second year of life and subsequently shows distinct developmental trajectories in different individuals.[4] Aggression is a problem which is present from early childhood, arguably from toddlerhood and perhaps from birth. Violence ultimately signals the failure of normal developmental processes to deal with something (*aggression*) that occurs naturally.[5] With this in mind, it will be important when assessing an individual's risk of violence to consider their developmental pathway. This will have influenced their potential for destructiveness as a result of an inability to manage aggressive impulses. Rutter et al (2001) showed that environmental influences that divert the child from paths of violence and behavioural disturbance often imply the establishment of strong attachment relationships with relatively healthy individuals.[6] The common pathway to violence is the momentary inhibition of the capacity for communication or for interpretation. It probably could not arise if early experience has built an interpersonal interpretive capacity of sufficient robustness to withstand later maltreatment.[7]

The requirement to explore the nature of attachments during all phases of childhood is central to the understanding of pathways towards violence within individuals. For a patient in whom there has been a failure of the development of secure attachments, a warning bell should ring in the clinician's mind. As well as the requirement to consider pathways from a developmental perspective, it is also necessary to consider other pathways leading to the violent act. These will include cultural issues (cultural traditions of violence especially) as well as a history of substance abuse and past episodes of violence.

Whilst considering these matters, it should not be forgotten that aggression is also a positive trait which throughout evolution has ensured survival in the context of threat and that it is still relevant today as an adaptive component of the human psyche.

There has been substantial discussion in the literature about whether mental illness does increase the risk of violence and, currently, the consensus seems to be that there is a slightly increased risk but it is small.[8,9,10]

Early work on the risk of violence in the mentally ill focussed mostly on its prediction and was carried out predominantly in forensic settings. Inquiries into homicide by persons with mental illness found that only a minority of incidents were predictable. Despite this, the majority could have been prevented with good risk management.[11,12] Current recommendations are that the only ethical justification for the assessment of the risk of violence is when risk reduction through risk management is also included.[13] The two areas in psychiatry in which violence has been studied most intensively are for those patients suffering from schizophrenia and for those patients with personality disorders, especially psychopathy. The trends which are emerging from the study of these two areas are likely to be applicable to other disorders.

BOX 15.1 AGGRESSION AND VIOLENCE: SUMMARY

- Aggression is a normal component of human functioning.
- Violence can be seen as the inability to control aggression or the use of aggression for personal gain.
- Failure to develop secure attachments is a risk factor for violence.
- Some cultures have a tradition of greater use of violence. It is necessary to factor this into history taking.
- Mental illness causes a slight increase in the risk of violence.

Risk factors for violence not always associated with mental illness

Many non-psychiatric variables, especially a combination of youth, male gender, substance use and low socioeconomic status, reveal a far greater association with violence than does mental illness.[14] Applying risk factors, especially static ones, in an unthinking way should be avoided. Simply to assume that maleness, for example, will lead to violence is not helpful. In the debate about which static risk factors to include in standardised rating scales, it is pertinent to note that male gender and youth have been left out of the Historical/Clinical/Risk Management 20-item (HCR 20) scale. The risk factors of most relevance in helping predict the *future, longer-term risk* of violence are those not necessarily associated with mental illness: the two most important static factors being substance misuse[15,16] and a past history of violence.[17] Drugs and alcohol are strongly associated with violent behaviour.[18] The majority of persons involved in violent crimes are under the influence of alcohol at the time of their aggression.[19] At least half of all violent events, including murders, were preceded by alcohol consumption by the perpetrator of a crime, the victim or both.[20] Stimulants which increase aggressiveness, grandiosity and paranoia, such as amphetamines and cocaine, are of special concern. Among psychiatric patients, a coexisting diagnosis of substance abuse is strongly predictive of violence.[21]

BOX 15.2 RISK FACTORS FOR VIOLENCE — NON MENTAL ILLNESS

- Most violence is perpetrated by those who are *not* mentally ill.
- Substance abuse and a past history of violence are the two most important static risk factors for violence.
- Alcohol and stimulants are the two drug groups most implicated when violence occurs.
- A detailed history of past episodes of violence is a prerequisite of an assessment of risk of violence.

Schizophrenia and violence

For violent behaviour, reports typically find that schizophrenia is related to a 4–6-fold increased risk of violent behaviour, which has led to the view that schizophrenia and other major mental disorders are preventable causes of violence and violent crime.[22] There has been considerable uncertainty about what mediates this elevated risk. Studies have begun to characterise a subpopulation of patients with schizophrenia whose course of illness and treatment is shaped by a complex developmental trajectory — the intertwining of psychosis with the sequelae of childhood antisocial conduct, trauma, victimisation and substance abuse. At the centre of this knot of pathologies lies the problem of violent behaviour.[23] Violence among adults with schizophrenia may follow two distinct pathways — one associated with premorbid conditions, including antisocial conduct, and the other associated with the acute psychopathology of schizophrenia.[24] For some time, it was felt that violence was predominantly mediated by the active symptoms of illness — mostly psychosis,[25] but more recently it appears that the association of schizophrenia and violence disappears when substance abuse is accounted for.[26] Similarly, if there is a history of conduct disorder, the likelihood of violence in schizophrenia is greater.[27] However, positive psychotic symptoms have been linked to violence in a group without conduct problems.[28]

Regarding homicide, there is some evidence of an increased risk in patients suffering from schizophrenia. In Shaw's paper from 2006, a rate of schizophrenia of 5% (lifetime) was found out of 1594 people convicted of homicide over a 3-year period.[29]

BOX 15.3 CLINICAL TIP

- Patients with a history of violence who stop medications or fail to attend follow-up sessions should generate an intervention. It should be clearly documented in both the treatment plan and the risk plan.
- Does your health board have a guideline/procedure or policy about this?

Psychosis and violence

Although the literature on this subject can be confusing at times, there is general, clinical consensus that acute symptoms of illness, mostly psychosis, are linked to an increased risk of violence.[30]

Delusions noted to increase the risk of violence are those characterised by having 'threat/control override' (TCO) symptoms.[31] These involve the following characteristics:

- that the mind is dominated by forces beyond the person's control
- that thoughts are being put into the person's head
- that people are wishing the person harm
- that the person is being followed.

Also, when delusional beliefs make subjects unhappy, frightened, anxious or angry, they are more likely to act aggressively. Non-delusional suspiciousness, such as misperceiving others' behaviour as indicating hostile intent, is also associated with subsequent violence.[32] A propensity to act on delusions in general is significantly associated with a tendency to commit violent acts.[33]

In general, the presence of hallucinations is not related to dangerous acts but in patients with schizophrenia; they are more likely to be violent if their hallucinations generate negative emotions such as anger, anxiety or sadness. The risk of violence is also greater if the patient has not developed successful strategies to cope with their voices.[34] There is a relationship between command hallucinations to commit violence and actual violence.[35] Lack of insight is also important.[36]

In the assessment, an attempt should be made to link symptoms with behaviour. Delusions and hallucinations are obviously important, but over-arousal, disinhibition and extremes of fear or anger are probably more common links between mental disorder and violence.[37]

BOX 15.4 VIOLENCE AND PSYCHOSIS: SUMMARY

- A past history of violence and/or substance abuse is of more predictive value than a history of psychosis.
- A childhood history of conduct disorder and/or failure of attachments is of substantial importance.
- Psychosis leading to fear, anger, over arousal and other emotional states is likely to be a common link between mental disorder and violence.
- Psychosis which is perceived by the patient as threatening and leads to a decision to 'override' normal inhibitory controls is of importance.
- A tendency to act on delusions is linked to violence.
- Command hallucinations to commit violence are a risk factor.
- There are likely to be two pathways leading to violence: one associated with premorbid conditions and the other with acute symptoms.
- Non-compliance with medication putting the patient at risk of a relapse of psychosis is of great importance.

Personality disorders and violence

The most common personality disorder associated with violence is anti-social personality disorder (ASPD).[38] However, this may be misleading as the majority of the research on personality disorders and violence has been carried out using the concept of psychopathy and especially the Hare Psychopathy Checklist, Revised (PCL-R).[39] There is an important difference between these two diagnoses. ASPD is predominantly based on behavioural manifestations whilst psychopathy utilises inter-personal, affective, lifestyle and antisocial constructs.[40] The construct of psychopathy does not exist within either DSM IV[41] or ICD 10,[42] which creates further problems for clinicians.

The interpersonal and affective components are seen as being central features to the construct of psychopathy. It is wrong to equate research on the risk of violence in psychopathy to violence in a patient with a diagnosis of ASPD. The diagnosis of ASPD is much more common than that of psychopathy and occurs approximately three times more frequently.[43] Similar arguments can be made between the diagnosis of dis-social personality disorder (ICD-10) and psychopathy.[44] Although the PCL-R and the Psychopathy Checklist: Screening Version (PCL: SV) are among the best predictors of risk for offending and risk for violence in psychiatric patients,[45] contemporary approaches to risk assessment require that these measures are not employed in isolation.[46] The rate of psychopathy in psychiatric populations is very low (i.e. approximately 1–2%) but it is important to emphasise the strong predictive quality of the Hare Psychopathy Checklist.[47] Unfortunately, using the Hare Psychopathy Checklist requires training and experience in psycho-pathology, psychometric assessment and the research in the field of psychopathy. However, knowledge of the findings from this work can be useful in everyday assessments.

The violence perpetrated by those with psychopathy is often moti-vated by revenge or occurs during a period of heavy drinking. Violence amongst these persons is frequently cold and calculated and lacks emo-tion.[48] The differentiation between affective and predatory violence[47] is a useful one to make. Affective aggression involves hostile behaviour as a reaction to some perceived threat, either from the environment or from an internal sense of fear or anxiety. In contrast, predatory aggres-sion is planned, purposeful and goal directed. Here the individual seeks a target to harm.[50] Predatory violence is more dangerous because there is usually an absence of observable antecedent behaviours that fore-shadow the aggression.[51]

Within a mental health setting, traits of personality disorders can emerge with the onset or a relapse of different illnesses. For example, a patient with mania or schizophrenia can present with features of ASPD or psychopathy whilst suffering from an acute relapse of their illness. This becomes important in risk management as the features of personal-ity disorder can at times lead clinicians to forget or ignore the aspects of their Axis I illness and miss out on some of the important risk factors. At its worst, the patient may be misdiagnosed as having a personality disorder and the Axis I disorder is missed entirely. (Personality disor-ders are classified under Axis II in the DSM IV multi-axial classifica-tion system.[52] Axis I disorders, which include major mental disorders, should always be considered.) In a similar vein, patients are sometimes misdiagnosed as having a drug-induced psychosis when any substance abuse is noted, which can lead to pejorative, stigmatised approaches by clinicians who then mismanage both the underlying illness and the risk issues.

Other disorders and violence

Depression may result in violent behaviour under certain circum-stances. For example, individuals who are depressed may strike out against others in despair. After committing a violent act, the depressed person may attempt suicide; for example, the psychotically depressed

BOX 15.5 VIOLENCE AND PERSONALITY DISORDERS: SUMMARY

- Violence is strongly linked with the diagnosis of psychopathy.
- In these patients, the violence is often cold and calculated and lacks emotion.
- In these patients, the violence is often motivated by revenge or occurs during a period of heavy drinking.
- Violence in patients with a diagnosis of psychopathy is often associated with predatory aggression which is planned, purposeful and goal directed. There is usually an absence of observable antecedent behaviour and the violence is targeted usually at one individual.
- Impulsive violence is more commonly a problem in ASPD compared to the planned violence seen in psychopathy.
- Patients who present with features of personality disorders during an onset or relapse of mental illness should not be treated as if the personality disorder was the primary problem. Active treatment of the Axis I disorder may often lead to the features of personality disorder resolving.

patient who kills his family and then himself. A very important subgroup of depressed patients is those with post-natal depression. There is a small percentage of these patients who develop psychotic symptoms and an even smaller subgroup who develop thoughts of killing their baby (infanticide). This small but significant group of patients need careful and skilled assessment and monitoring.

Morbid jealousy has long been recognised as being a risk factor for violence.

Patients with mania show a high percentage of assaulting or threatening behaviour, but serious violence itself is rare.[53]

Post-traumatic stress disorder (PTSD) is frequently a response to extreme violence. Some of the symptoms of PTSD — anger, hypervigilance and hyper-arousal — may be triggered by stimuli which remind the patient of the initial trauma. For some patients, the stimuli may be relatively minor, but may spark off a fight/flight response which in some situations may lead to violence. This is especially the case if the trigger is a person who reminds the patient of the perpetrator of the initial trauma. The patient may then enter a dissociative state and perceive themselves as needing to fight for their lives.

Brain injury or illness should also be considered as a risk factor for aggressive and violent behaviour. After a brain injury or in a delirious state, formerly peaceful individuals may become verbally or physically aggressive. Depending on the site of the injury, patients may lose normal capacity to perceive and process a threat. Impulse controls may have disappeared as a result of the brain injury. For some brain injuries, especially in the amygdala, aggression may be greater than prior to the injury. (The amygdala, part of the limbic system, performs a primary role in the processing and memory of emotional reactions.) In frontal lobe injuries, violence may no longer be linked to shame, guilt or other inhibitory mechanisms that would have been previously present in a patient.

BOX 15.6 VIOLENCE AND OTHER DISORDERS: SUMMARY

- Violence associated with strong affect is often linked to some perceived threat, either from the environment or from an internal sense of fear or anxiety.
- Many psychiatric disorders will be associated with strong affects, including fear, anger, heightened levels of arousal and increased impulsivity. The likelihood of violence will be increased in these circumstances.
- Organic brain disorders may also cause similar disturbance of affective control.

As can be seen from this brief review, the research into static factors for violence is more comprehensive and, indeed, is the focus of most rating scales. The problem of dynamic factors for violence is less well researched but is arguably of more interest and importance to clinicians working at the coalface. Dynamic risk factors are harder to elucidate from a research perspective but, nevertheless, clinicians should be able to utilise current knowledge in their everyday work to identify which dynamic factors are of importance in individual patients. The next problem is that, as was the case for the static factors, some dynamic factors for violence are not necessarily related to mental illness. Impulsivity, antisocial attitudes, current substance abuse and breakdown of interpersonal relationships are all dynamic factors which may occur in the absence of mental illness.

Other important dynamic factors which are related to mental illness, but not specific disorders, are those of non-compliance with medication, poor treatment-provider alliance and having a treatment plan which is not likely to work.

The following list of dynamic risk factors has been proposed for research purposes.[54] It is made up from a list of the leading risk factors for violence and they have been selected as they are malleable; that is, they can change with relevant treatment.

Proposed dynamic risk factors
- Impulsiveness
- Negative affectivity
  - anger
  - negative mood
- Psychosis
- Antisocial attitudes
- Substance use and related problems
- Interpersonal relationships
- Treatment alliance and adherence
  - treatment and medication compliance
  - treatment/provider alliance

This list covers most of the factors that have been highlighted in the summary boxes. It is necessary to remember that the proposed negative affects would include fear and hyper-arousal. Similarly, it does not elaborate on the specific contents of psychosis which have been discussed and these also need to be remembered. In the summary of risk factors for violence at the end of the chapter (Table 15.1), the static, dynamic and protective factors have been laid out in a form which can be printed on an A4 sheet and used as an aide memoire in the clinical situation. All the risk factors highlighted are included.

Screening for assessment for risk of violence

The decision about when to undertake a full assessment of violence is difficult to make. *Imminent risk* of violence may be mediated and predicted by acute psychiatric symptoms, often in the context of substance use.[55,56] It is important to remember that a history of substance use helps predict both future risk and long-term risk, and current substance use helps predict imminent risk.

A screening tool was developed at the Institute of Psychiatry, London, in 2002[57] and may be useful in helping clinicians during an assessment to make a decision about whether to undertake a full risk assessment and management plan. The screening tool forms Figure 15.1.

This screening tool could be used to guide clinicians at times of uncertainty. For certain patients — inpatients, forensic patients — a risk assessment and management plan will automatically be generated, but at other times, these prompts may be of use.

Table 15.1 Risk factors for violence

Risk factors for violence

Static factors

- Male gender and younger age of first violent incident.
- Past history of violence. Consider the degree of violence and the frequency.
- Substance use. Is this historical and/or is it continuing today?
- Childhood maladjustments and behavioural problems and childhood abuse.

Nature of the risk

- Risk to whom, type of weapon? Well formulated or poorly developed plans?
- Predatory or affective type of violence?

Illness (dynamic) factors

- Psychosis — is the patient threatened, frightened and are normal controls overridden?
- Does the patient feel persecuted?
- Is the patient having command hallucinations?
- Changing symptoms. A tendency to act on symptoms.
- Impulsivity. Lack of insight.
- Violent thoughts being expressed? Morbid jealousy?
- Threatening or fearful behaviour.
- Current diagnosis of personality disorder — especially psychopathy but include antisocial personality disorder.
- Self-report of thoughts of violence.

Situational factors

- Current substance use.
- Unstable accommodation. Unemployed. Current stressors.
- Poor compliance with medication. Poor therapeutic alliance.
- Access to weapons.

Protective factors

- What has worked previously to prevent violence?
- Good therapeutic alliance.
- Family support?
- Concern about harming others. Awareness of triggers.

Continued

Table 15.1 Risk factors for violence—cont'd

Risk factors for violence

Systemic factors

- Do carers think there is a problem?
- Is the situation at home deteriorating?
- Is the treatment plan feasible?

Early warning signs and triggers

- What has helped in the past?
- Does the patient have good or poor insight into his/her illness?
- Can the patient recognise their triggers?

Relapse indicators

- Does the patient or their carers recognise indicators of relapse?
- Will the patient accept treatment voluntarily?

Current thoughts, plans or symptoms indicating a risk of violence?	Y/N
Current behaviour suggesting there is a risk of violence?	Y/N
Current problems with alcohol or substance abuse?	Y/N
Significant past history of violence?	Y/N
Expression of concern from others about risk of violence?	Y/N

After taking into account other relevant information and the extent to which information is available to you after the final screening question:

In your professional judgment, is a full assessment of risk of violence indicated?   Y/N

(Source: Reproduced with permission from Watts D, Bindman J, Slade M, Holloway F, Rosen A, Thornicroft G 2004 Clinical assessment of risk decision support (CARDS): the development and evaluation of a feasible violence riskassessment for routine psychiatric practice. *Journal of Mental Health,*13 (6):569-81.

Figure 15.1 Screening tool for risk of violence

As described elsewhere in this book, the best form of assessment is considered to be structured clinical judgment,[58] using a narrative approach.[59] In forensic settings, standardised assessment tools are often used to help develop objective risk assessments, monitor treatment, assist in discharge planning and in the development of risk management plans. More recently, scales have been developed to predict violence in inpatient settings. The scales have not focused on any one particular illness but have developed criteria which can be generalised to many acute situations. These are explored in more detail in Chapter 18.

Obtaining a detailed violence history involves determining the type of violent behaviour, asking if weapons were used, why violence occurred, who was involved, the presence of intoxication and the degree of injury. Criminal and court records are particularly useful in evaluating the person's past history of violence and illegal behaviour. The age at first arrest for a serious offence is highly correlated with persistence of criminal offending.[60] Each prior episode of violence increases the risk of a future violent act.

Talking to the patient, relatives and caregivers

The potentially violent patient needs to know and understand why interventions are necessary. Asking a patient about violence has not been shown to increase the likelihood of a violent act occurring and helps establish rapport. Questions about the triggers for violence and a patient's feelings about being violent give vital information.[61] Asking about fantasies, plans to harm others, access to weapons, capacity for self-control and their feelings for their victims adds further important information.[62]

Violence involves others. Relatives and caregivers often complain of aspects of the patient's behaviour which, though not involving physical violence, produce fear and distress. All too often this fear-inducing behaviour is dismissed, or minimised, by mental health professionals. Emergence of irritability and threatening and scary behaviours is frequently the way that relapse into delusions and psychotic experiences declares itself.[63] Violence is the endpoint of a series of external and internal events. The final releasing factor for the violent event will, of course, vary from person to person, but of immense importance is the risk factors which can be identified, especially critical risk factors unique to the individual. Working with the patient to identify the tipping point for violence is perhaps the central task of the risk assessment and management of violence.

Some patients will continue to behave violently for reasons not felt to be related to their illness or to their treatment. Sometimes this will be driven by psychopathy which is not felt to be treatable in an inpatient setting. At other times there will be discussion about whether the violence is driven by factors such as substance abuse which may be

BOX 15.7 CLINICAL TIP

- If a family member phones and says that they have become frightened about your patient, take note. Fear expressed by the family is often the first indicator of a heightened risk of violence. This should be included in the risk management plan.
- Listening to relatives and other caregivers provides vital information which should not be ignored.

treatable but the patient may decline care. On these occasions, robust discussion within the multidisciplinary team (MDT), with the patient and with their family will often help in clarifying the next step. Utilising a risk/benefit analysis with all concerned can also help. The ethical and moral considerations should be discussed at these times. The guidance of a senior staff member/team leader who is not risk averse at these times is invaluable.

Exercise 1 — identifying personal signals for danger

Most of us have been in dangerous situations with patients. Do you know your personal signals which warn you that a similar situation is developing? What are they? In the following example, consider your personal triggers and when they might be pulled.

A 25-year-old man has been admitted to your inpatient ward overnight. You are a junior nurse and arrive at work for the morning shift. In handover, you are told that the patient has not been in hospital before and this is his first episode of illness. The events leading up to his admission were that he had been picked up in the main street of town having been wandering in an aimless, somewhat confused way at 3 a.m. When the police asked him if he was all right, he looked at them in a perplexed, bewildered way and they took him to the Emergency Department (ED). The admitting team felt that he was probably psychotic but as he is virtually mute, it is difficult to determine this. As yet, it has not been possible to contact his family. In the handover meeting, the team decides that the best plan is to try and engage the young man as far as possible, make him comfortable and see if he can be persuaded to talk a little bit more. You are allocated to be his primary nurse.

During the course of the day, you feel as if you make minimal headway. The patient remains uncommunicative but does respond to his name and also when asked to undertake simple tasks such as going to the dining room for a meal, etc. As the shift progresses, you find yourself becoming a little bit uncomfortable and almost frightened in his presence and try and work out why you are feeling this. You note that his eye contact has changed and he now seems to stare at you more intensely. He has begun to pace the corridor and is watching the doorway. Other than this, there are no particular indicators that you can put your finger on, but he seems to become less willing to follow simple directions. On reflection, he reminds you of a similar patient who was violent on the ward 3 months ago. At the end of the shift, you share your concerns with the new staff coming on duty. They apply the Dynamic Appraisal of Situational Aggression (DASA) scale [64] (see Chapter 18, page 191) during their shift and this is repeated on a daily basis. The scores are used to help address the management of the potential risk of violence. As he becomes more communicative, the patient starts to become verbally threatening for a few days, but then this settles. On one occasion he hit the wall with his fist for no apparent reason. When he is able to tell you what was happening, he says that he was very frightened as he felt that he was going to be attacked because of his religious beliefs but could not work out who was going to attack him. He knew that he would have to defend himself if anybody got too close.

Refer to Appendix 3 for a discussion of this exercise.

More prompts and interviewing questions in greater detail can be found in:

- New Zealand Ministry of Health 2006 Assessment and Management of Risk to Others Guidelines; Development of Training Toolkit; and Trainee Workbook. New Zealand Ministry of Health. Online. Available: www.mhwd.govt.nz
- Institute of Psychiatry, London 2002 CARDS assessment guidelines. Health Services Research Department, Institute of Psychiatry, London. Online. Available: www.iop.kcl.ac.uk/iopweb/virtual/?path=/hsr/prism/cards/

Notes

1 Mullen PE 1997 A reassessment of the link between mental disorder and violent behaviour, and its implications for clinical practice. *Australian and New Zealand Journal of Psychiatry*, 31:3–11.

2 De Zulueta F 1993 *From Pain to Violence: the Traumatic Roots of Destructiveness.* Whurr Publishers, London.

3 Maden A 2007 *Treating Violence: a Guide to Risk Management in Mental Health.* Oxford University Press, Oxford.

4 Nagin DS, Tremblay RE 2001 Parental and early childhood predictors of persistent physical aggression in boys from kindergarten to high school. *Archives of Gen Psychiatry*, 58:389–94.

5 Fonagy P 2003 Towards a developmental understanding of violence. *British Journal of Psychiatry*, 183:190–2.

6 Rutter M, Pickles A, Murray R et al 2001 Testing hypotheses on specific environmental causal effects on behaviour. *Psychological Bulletin*, 127:291–324.

7 Fonagy, above, n 5.

8 Mullen, above, n 1.

9 Brennan PA, Grekin ER, Vanman EJ 2000 Major mental disorders and crime in the community. In: Hodgins S (ed.) *Violence Among the Mentally Ill*, Kluver Academic Publishers, Dordrecht.

10 Arsenault L, Caspi A, Moffitt TE et al 2000 Mental disorders and violence in a total birth cohort. *Archives of General Psychiatry*, 57:979–86.

11 Munro E, Rumgay J 2000 Role of risk assessment in reducing homicides by people with mental illness. *British Journal of Psychiatry*, 2:116–20.

12 Simpson AI, Allnut S, Chaplow D 2001 Inquiries into homicides and serious violence perpetrated by psychiatric patients in New Zealand: need for consistency of method and result analysis. *Australian and New Zealand Journal of Psychiatry*, 35:364–9.

13 Kumar S, Simpson AI 2005 Application of risk assessment for violence methods to general adult psychiatry: a selected literature review. *Australian and New Zealand Journal of Psychiatry*, 39:328–35.

14 Turner T 2008 Forensic psychiatry and general psychiatry: re-examining the relationship. *Psychiatric Bulletin*, 32:2–6.

15 Roth JA 1994 *Psychoactive Substance and Violence*. Online. Available: www.druglibrary.org/schaffer/GovPubs/PSYCVIOL.HTM (accessed 30 Nov 2009).

16 Norko M, Baranoski MV 2005 In review, the state of contemporary risk assessment research. *Canadian Journal of Psychiatry*, 50:18–26.

17 MacArthur Foundation 2001 *The MacArthur violence risk assessment study executive summary*. Online. Available: www.macarthur.virginia.edu/risk.html (accessed 11 Aug 2002).

18 MacArthur Foundation, above, n 17.

19 Murdoch D, Pihl RO, Ross D 1990 Alcohol and crimes of violence: present issues. *International Journal of the Addictions*, 25:1065–81.

20 Roth, above, n 15.

21 MacArthur Foundation, above, n 17.

22 Joyal C, Dubreucq J-L, Grendon C, Millaud F 2007 Major mental disorders and violence: a critical update. *Curr Psychiatry Review*, 3:33–50.

23 Swanson J, Van Dorn R, Swartz M, Smith A, Elbogen E, Monahan J 2008 Alternative pathways to violence in persons with schizophrenia: the role of childhood antisocial behaviour problems. *Law Hum Behav*, 32:228–40.

24 Swanson et al, above, n 23.

25 Link BG, Andrews H, Cullen FT 1992 The violent and illegal behaviour of mental patients reconsidered. *American Sociological Review*, 57:275–92.

26 Fazel S, Langstrom N, Hjern A, Grann M, Lichtenstein P 2009 Schizophrenia, substance abuse, and violent crime. *Journal of the American Medical Association*, 301(19):2016–23.

27 Hodgins S, Tiihonen J, Ross D 2005 The consequences of conduct disorder for males to develop schizophrenia: Associations with criminality, aggressive behaviour, substance use and psychiatric services. *Schizophrenia Research*, 78:323–35.

28 Swanson et al, above, n 23.

29 Shaw J, Hunt IM, Flynn S, Meehan J, Robinson J, Bickley H, Parsons R, McCann K, Burns J, Amos T, Kapur N, Appleby L 2006 Rates of mental disorder in people convicted of homicide: a national clinical survey. *British Journal of Psychiatry*, 188:143–7.

30 Scott CL, Resnick PJ 2006 Violence risk assessment in persons with mental illness. *Aggression and Violent Behaviour*, 11:598–611.

31 Link et al, above, n 25.

32 Monahan J, Henry J, Applebaum PS, Robbins PC, Mulvey EP, Silver EA, et al 2000 Developing a clinically useful actuarial tool for assessing violence risk. *British Journal of Psychiatry*, 176:312–9.

33 Monahan et al, above, n 32.

34 Cheung P, Schweitzer I, Crowley K, Tuckwell V 1997 Violence and schizophrenia: role of hallucinations and delusions. *Schizophrenia Research*, 26:181–90.

35 MacArthur Foundation, above, n 17.

36 Buckley PF, Hrouda DR, Friedman L, Noffsinger SG, Resnick PJ, Camlin-Shinger K 2004 Insight and its relationship to violent behaviour in patients with schizophrenia. *American Journal of Psychiatry*, 161:1712–14.

37 Maden A 1996 Risk assessment in psychiatry. *British Journal Hospital Medicine*, 56:78–82.

38 MacArthur Foundation, above, n 17.

39 Hare RD 2003 *Manual for the Hare Psychopathy Checklist* (2nd edn, revised). Multi-Health Systems, Toronto.

40 Ogloff JRP 2006 Psychopathy/antisocial personality disorder conundrum. *Australian and New Zealand Journal of Psychiatry* 40:519–28.

41 American Psychiatric Association 2000 *Diagnostic and Statistical Manual of Mental Disorders* (DSM IV TR). American Psychiatric Association.

42 World Health Organization 1990 *International Classification of Diseases* (ICD 10). World Health Organization, Geneva.

43 Cunningham MP, Reidy TJ 1998 Antisocial PD and psychopathy: diagnostic dilemmas in classifying patterns of antisocial behaviour in sentencing evaluations. *Behavioural Sciences and the Law*, 16:333–51.

44 Ogloff, above, n 40.

45 Nicholls TL, Ogloff JRP, Douglas KS 2004 Assessing risk for violence among male and female civil psychiatric patients: the HCR-20, PCL: SV, and McNeil and Binder's screening measure. *Behavioural Sciences and the Law*, 22:127–58.

46 Ogloff JRP, Davis MR 2005 Assessing risk for violence in the Australian context. In: Chapel D, Wilson P (eds) *Crime and Justice in the New Millennium*, Lexis Nexis, Sydney, pp 301–38.

47 Ogloff, above, n 40.

48 Williamson F, Hare RD, Wong S 1987 Violence: Criminal psychopaths and their victims. *Canadian Journal of Behavioural Science*, 19:454–62.

49 Meloy JR 1987 The prediction of violence in outpatient psychotherapy. *American Journal of Psychotherapy*, 41:38–45.

50 Scott and Resnick, above, n 30.

51 Meloy, above, n 47.

52 American Psychiatric Association, above, n 41.

53 Krakowski M, Volavka J, Brizer D 1986 Psychopathology and violence: a review of literature. *Comprehensive Psychiatry*, 27:131–48.

54 Douglas KS, Skeem JL 2005 Violence risk assessment. Getting specific about being dynamic. *Psychology, Public Policy and Law*, 11(3):347–83.

55 Norko and Baranoski, above, n 16.

56 McNeil DE, Gregory AL, Lam JN, Binder RL, Sullivan GR 2003 Utility of decision support tools for assessing acute risk of violence. *J Consult Clin Psychol*, 71:945–53.

57 Watts D, Bindman J, Slade M, Holloway F, Rosen A, Thornicroft G 2004 Clinical assessment of risk decision support (CARDS): the development and evaluation of a feasible violence risk assessment for routine psychiatric practice. *Journal of Mental Health*, 13(6):569–81.

58 Monahan J, Steadman HJ, Silver EA, Applebaum PS (eds) 2001 *Rethinking Risk Assessment: the MacArthur Study of Mental Disorder and Violence*, Oxford Press, New York.

59 Higgins N, Watts D, Bindman J, Slade M, Thornicroft G 2005 Assessing violence risk in general adult psychiatry. *Psychiatric Bulletin*, 29:131–3.

60 Borum R, Swartz M, Swanson J 1996 Assessing and managing violence risk in clinical practice. *Journal of Practical Psychiatry and Behavioural Health*, 4:205–15.

61 Kumar and Simpson, above, n 13.

62 Litwack TR 2001 Actuarial versus clinical assessment of dangerousness. *Psychology, Public Policy, and Law*, 7:409–43.

63 Mullen, above, n 1.

64 Ogloff JRP, Daffern M 2003 *The Assessment of Inpatient Aggression at the Thomas Embling Hospital: Towards the Dynamic Appraisal of Inpatient Aggression*. Forensicare, Victorian Institute of Forensic Mental Health Fourth Annual Research Report to Council, 1 July 2002–30 June 2003.

PART 4

ADVANCED SKILLS

16 Psychodynamic principles and boundaries

> However much he loves his patients he cannot avoid hating them, and the better he knows this, the less will hate and fear be the motives determining what he does to his patients.[1]

The quote above is from Winnicott (1949): on likening the care for the psychotic or difficult patient to a mother caring for a demanding baby.

Psychodynamics can be simply described as the understanding and study of the conscious and unconscious motivations that underlie human behaviour. They can be explored from the perspective of the individual's psychological functioning and from the interaction between people and groups of people. This brief chapter provides a glimpse into the role that psychodynamic principles can have in risk assessment and management. A psychodynamic contribution to risk assessment adds information which cannot be obtained from standardised rating scales, but which can be of use in understanding the meaning and function of the risk behaviour for the patient. As well as exploring the psychological functioning of the patient, this contribution looks at the *interaction* between the therapist, the patient and others involved. It examines the therapist's responses and it allows for a more meaningful interpretation and understanding of the risk behaviour. Ultimately this will lead to a more useful formulation of the risk and how it can be explained in the context of the patient's illness, their interaction with their friends and family, and also their interaction with health professionals.

Taking a psychodynamic approach to the clinical presentation allows for an explanation of the mechanisms driving the risk behaviour. Risk behaviours (e.g. violence, suicidality, etc.) usually occur when an affect fails to be contained, regulated or linked to other mental mechanisms by thinking. Repetitive risk behaviours can be explored using the concept of repetition compulsion (see glossary). Past acts can be explored to discover their meaning for the patient and their continuing function in the here and now.

> It is important to gain an understanding of the patient's risk from the inside: understanding what the patient's attitude to the behaviour is. Try to understand how the world is viewed through the patient's eyes.[2]

Considering the following questions will help develop understanding of the risk behaviour which simple exploration of the risk factors will miss.

- Does the patient express regret or remorse for the victim?
- Does the patient have capacity for empathy?
- Why has this particular person been chosen as the potential recipient of violence?
- Is there a theme to the patient's self-harm or violence?
- Does the patient's risk behaviour have an effect on particular staff? If so, what is the effect and why does it happen?
- Does the patient's risk behaviour make sense in the light of the patient's developmental history and life events?

Certain types of risk tend to promote more fear or rescuing behaviour on the part of some clinicians. To understand this involves an exploration of the transference and counter-transference (see glossary). What information does this give the clinician about the nature of the risk for the patient?

Asking questions about fantasy will give further information which may help make sense of the risk behaviour, especially violence and sexual risks. For patients with chronic risk, a central theme of the treatment is an exploration of the emotions and cognitions driving the behaviour. For patients with 'time-based and contingent suicidal intent'[3] (see page 137), the proposed date of death is a communication whose meaning needs to be explored before it can be managed.

Psychodynamic approaches can also be used to explore individual and group responses to perceived risk. Fear, anxiety, anger, panic, denial and so forth can be considered at both an individual and a group level. Individually, a clinician may reflect on their own practice but can also use supervision and second opinions. In a team which is functioning healthily, group discussions will be facilitated by the team leader and will help reduce the likelihood of a collective abuse of emotional responses. Other group responses to perceived risk, such as rejection, scapegoating, malignant alienation,[4] victimisation, prejudice, stigma and so forth, can also be explored with good facilitation by the team leader.[5]

With experience, clinicians begin to recognise counter-transferential responses in certain types of clinical situations and, as the likelihood of acting on them reduces, these responses can be utilised as tools both in helping to make the diagnosis but also to assist in exploring the meaning of the risk.

The following exercises are very brief vignettes which are designed to demonstrate common clinical scenarios in which an emotional response on the part of the clinician is likely to occur. Many clinicians will have anecdotal stories where the emotions on the day affected good clinical management — focussing on psychodynamic principles should reduce this risk.

Exercise 1 — Sonny

You're asked to assess a man, Sonny, with severe alcohol dependence. He has two convictions for assault on women. You know that female staff feel uncomfortable in his presence. He is involved with a female patient, younger than him, who has an opiate dependence. You are asked as the male/female staff member to assess his risk of future assaults and propose management. How does a psychodynamic approach to risk assessment add value to the overall assessment of risk?

Refer to Appendix 3 for discussion of this exercise.

Exercise 2 — Julie

Julie is 24, has borderline personality disorder (BPD) and self-harms frequently by cutting her wrists deeply and taking overdoses. At the time of self-harming, she says that she wants to die, but a day later she says that she just wanted a break from the torment. Your supervisor asks you to consider how a psychodynamic approach to the assessment of risk may add meaning to the behaviours from the perspective of the family, the patient and staff caring for her.

Refer to Appendix 3 for discussion of this exercise.

Exercise 3 — Harry (scapegoating?)

Harry has schizophrenia, is quite insightful and is treated pharmacologically with olanzapine. He has ongoing positive symptoms of command hallucinations. At the MDT, a case manager feels that he would benefit from clozapine but the consultant disagrees. The case manager fears that Harry will act on his hallucinations and kill someone. As team leader, you know that the consultant is apprehensive about using clozapine as a patient of his had a close call with a low white cell count recently. As team leader, how do you manage the risk?

Refer to Appendix 3 for discussion of this exercise.

> ## BOX 16.1 PSYCHODYNAMIC PRINCIPLES
>
> **Practice points**
> - Using psychodynamic principles can add depth and meaning to the risk assessment.
> - Psychodynamic principles can be used to help understand individual and group responses to risk.

Boundary issues

Boundaries in mental health settings usually refer to the rules, written and unwritten, that guide the professional relationship between the patient and clinician. They can include issues relating to touching patients, divulging personal information, the acceptance of gifts, etc. Because therapeutic relationships use emotions, feelings, visual cues and so on as an integral component of treatment, the relationship can be exposed to risky behaviours if there are no clear boundaries. Clinicians need to be aware of their own emotional state, should not infect the therapeutic relationship with unresolved emotions of their own and need to guard against infection from the emotional states of their patients.

Using the emotional state of both the patient and the clinician to assist in the assessment and management of risk also exposes the clinician to the risk of mismanagement of their own emotions. Boundary indiscretions or violations are real risks to which all clinicians will be exposed on a regular basis if they are not able to manage their own emotional responses in the clinical situation. The personality style of the clinician should be taken into account when boundary issues are being considered. Different personality styles can work well for different patients. Some clinicians can manage patients with psychosis very much more easily than patients with personality disorders, and vice versa. The more conscious a clinician is of their own personality style the better the chance of reducing the likelihood of counter-transference problems intruding upon a therapeutic relationship.

Some clinicians choose to suppress their emotional response, which reduces the risk of a breach of boundaries but also limits the opportunities to use the interpersonal relationship as a therapeutic tool. A common cause of difficulties leading to boundary violations is *projective identification*. In its simplest form, a patient projects an emotional state or belief onto their therapist unconsciously, because they are currently unable to incorporate it into their consciousness. For example, this may be an inability to express love. The therapist receives the projection of love and begins to behave (unconsciously acting out counter-transference) in a loving and caring way towards the patient beyond the usual levels of professional care. This process generally happens outside the awareness of both patient and therapist. As may be imagined, this can cause mayhem within treatment, but it can also be a cause of boundary violation. Counter-transference in its simplest form is the clinician's emotional response, which stems from both the specific relationship with the patient and the character and disposition of the clinician. When counter-transference is a conscious response, it can shed light on the patient's personality and ways of relating, but when unconscious it may give rise to well-rationalised but destructive acting out by the clinician.[6]

As described above, the counter-transferential responses of anxiety, fear, anger and love can all be used to assist in the assessment as well as the care of the patient, but if they are not conscious and managed by the clinician, they may be expressed within the therapeutic relationship inappropriately, will lead to poor outcomes and may well lead to a boundary violation. Crossing therapeutic boundaries is a problem which has been highlighted in the media, especially when there has been sexual contact with a patient. However, this is the most overt form of harm which is read about. The more subtle harms, often covert misuse of anger and reflexive responses to anxiety, are equally damaging and more pernicious. Equally destructive is the reflexive response, when faced with a difficult patient, of resorting to the moral high ground of rationality and the 'scientific attitude'.[7]

Boundary violations do not suddenly happen. A common sequence involves a transition from last-name to first-name basis, then personal conversation intruding on the clinical work, then some body contact (e.g. pats on the shoulder progressing to hugs), then sessions over lunch and finally sexual intercourse.[8]

Apart from the harm done to the patient, violation of boundaries is a serious type of professional misconduct which may lead to loss of professional license. Clinicians need to manage this risk proactively.

For more detailed explorations of this topic, suggested books are:

- Gabbard GO, Lester EP 2002 *Boundaries and Boundary Violations in Psychoanalysis*. American Psychiatric Publishing. Online. Available: http://appi.org/book.cfm?id=62098 (accessed 22 Nov 2009)
- Gutheil TG, Brodsky A 2008 *Preventing Boundary Violations in Clinical Practice*. The Guilford Press. Online. Available: http://www.guilford.com/cgi-bin/cartscript.cgi?page=pr/gutheil (accessed 22 Nov 2009)

Exercise 4 — boundary issues: John, Sarah and Lynley

For these hypothetical situations think about your emotional responses and how you might manage them.

1 John is 35 years old and presents with an impulse control disorder. He has a history of assaulting his girlfriends. You are also 35 years old, *male*, and your current girlfriend has had a troubled past in some of her relationships.

2 John is 35 years old and presents with an impulse control disorder. He has a history of assaulting his girlfriends. You are also 35 years old, *female*, and have been threatened by men in the past.

3 Sarah is 23 years old, self-harms, and presents in a slightly sexually provocative but also vulnerable and helpless way. You are:
    (a) a 50-year-old parent with a daughter of a similar age
    (b) 28 years old and find Sarah attractive.

4 Lynley is a 45-year-old woman with an anxiety disorder and dependent personality traits. You assess her as moderately depressed and feel that you can manage her within the home-based treatment team. Her family demand that she be admitted and say that if you refuse, they will complain to the ombudsman and go to the national newspapers.

Refer to Appendix 3 for a discussion of Exercise 4.

Questions to ask yourself when boundary issues are concerned:

- Are you maintaining your professional role? If in doubt, read your profession's code of conduct guidelines or ask a colleague.
- Are you maintaining good professional boundaries when you see your patients? Are you seeing them within clinic hours or after hours? Have you started seeing your patients during your lunch hour or over a cup of coffee?
- When transporting a patient, especially one of the opposite sex, do you have a colleague with you in the car?

BOX 16.2 BOUNDARY ISSUES

Practice points
- Emotional responses to risk situations can have a bearing on how the risk is managed.
- Creating a work environment which allows time for reflection will help reduce boundary violations.
- Discussion with colleagues and regular supervision further helps the exploration of emotional responses to risky situations.

- Have you considered issues of self-disclosure and physical contact in your practice?

If in doubt, discuss the issue with a colleague or your supervisor before undertaking any course of action.

Notes

1 Winnicott DW 1949 Hate in the counter-transference. *International Journal of Psychoanalysis*, 30:69–74.

2 Grounds A 1995 Risk assessment and management in clinical context. In: Crichton J (ed) *Psychiatric Patient Violence — Risk and Response*, Duckworth, London, pp 43–59.

3 Gutheil TG, Schetky D 1998 A date with death: management of time-based and contingent suicidal intent. *American Journal of Psychiatry*, 155:1502–7.

4 Watts D, Morgan HG 1994 Malignant alienation. Dangers for patients who are hard to like. *British Journal of Psychiatry*, 164:11–5.

5 Murphy D 2002 Risk assessment as collective clinical judgment. *Criminal Behaviour and Mental Health*, 12:169–78.

6 Doctor R 2004 Psychodynamic lessons in risk assessment and management. *Advances in Psychiatric Treatment*, 10:267–76.

7 Hinshelwood RD 1999 The difficult patient. The role of 'scientific psychiatry' in understanding patients with chronic schizophrenia or severe personality disorder. *British Journal of Psychiatry*, 174:187–90.

8 Gutheil TG, Gabbard GD 1993 The concept of boundaries in clinical practice: theoretical and risk management. *American Journal of Psychiatry*, 150:188–96.

17 Managing adverse outcomes

Adverse events usually originate at a variety of systemic levels: the patient–clinician interaction, the team, the working environment and the organisation. Consideration of all of these factors is required when investigating and preventing adverse outcomes. The liability to make an *error* is strongly affected by the context and conditions of work, and the chain of events leading to an adverse outcome is usually complex. The root cause may be in several interlocking factors such as the use of locums, communication problems, supervision problems, excessive workload, resource limitations and training deficiencies. Analysis of accidents/adverse outcomes in mental health should explore not just the individual factors but also pre-existing organisational factors.

This process of review is usually called a *root cause analysis*. Root cause analysis is defined as a systematic iterative process whereby the factors which contribute to an incident are identified by reconstructing the sequence of events and repeatedly asking 'why?' until the underlying root causes (contributing factors/hazards) have been elucidated. Once this has occurred, changes can be made to whichever systems were found to be problematic.

There are 2 types of errors leading to adverse outcomes:

1 active failures
2 latent failures.

Active failures

Active failures are those acts or omissions committed by individuals that have an immediate adverse consequence. Where possible, failsafe mechanisms are brought in to guard against human error; for example, sharps boxes or computerised prescribing programs that do not allow excessive doses to be prescribed. Active failures can be divided into three subgroups:

1 Action slips or failures, such as labelling the wrong blood sample. Departure from routine is a major factor in the absent-minded slips of action.[1]
2 Cognitive failures, such as memory lapses or making mistakes through ignorance.
3 Violations which are deviations from usual operating practice without good reason. These are more likely to occur secondary to low morale, poor modelling from senior staff or inadequate management.

Latent failures

Latent failures provide the conditions in which adverse events occur and are the responsibility of all clinicians and managers. They include:

- heavy workloads
- inadequate knowledge
- inadequate supervision
- stressful environment
- rapid change within an organisation
- inadequate systems of communication.

These are the factors that influence staff performance and may precipitate errors and affect patient outcomes. The process of latent failures increasing the likelihood of active failures can be shown diagrammatically (see Figure 17.1).[2] The latent failures are transmitted along various organisational and departmental pathways to the workplace where they create local conditions that precipitate errors and violations. This model creates a more complicated picture where the environment in which an adverse event occurs is one where many factors are added, one to another, before the accident happens. Minimising the likelihood

Latent failures	Conditions of work	Active failures	Barriers/ defences	Accident
Stressful environment. Inadequate knowledge. Organisational processes.	Background factors: <ul><li>workload</li><li>supervision</li><li>communication</li><li>equipment</li><li>ability.</li></ul>	Unsafe acts: <ul><li>action slips/ failures</li><li>cognitive failures (memory lapses and mistakes)</li><li>violations.</li></ul>		

Figure 17.1 **The multifactorial pathway to accidents**

of adverse events occurring requires attention at all these levels by all staff, from the most junior to the most senior.

For senior professional staff, the task of creating an environment where errors are reduced can seem daunting. Regular auditing of compliance with guidelines and procedures is a useful start. The presence of a risk management team for the mental health service can be of immense use. The risk management team can review incidents, compile themes of recurring incidents and look for causes of errors and adverse events. When this is given in the form of feedback to staff, the cycle of reviewing risk is complete. Reviews conducted sensitively, in an environment in which healthy enquiry and no blame occurs, enable staff to participate fully and make maximum use of the experience.

Reviews of this type can benefit from the use of reflective practice at a group level. Using John's[3] model or Rolfe's et al (2001)[4] and asking the questions within a group setting reduces the likelihood of blame occurring and can give a framework for exploring adverse outcomes.

Finally, a summary of error producing conditions ranked in order of increased likelihood of the event happening can be sobering (see Table 17.1).[5]

Rather than waiting for an adverse outcome, all mental health teams and mental health services should have an ongoing audit cycle asking questions about whether systems and processes are working. As a result of auditing, new procedures can be put in place which, hopefully, will reduce the likelihood of an adverse outcome. Despite best efforts, adverse outcomes will still occur. The immediate thought when adverse outcomes are considered is the death of a patient. However, adverse

Table 17.1 Ranked summary of error producing conditions

Condition	Risk factor
Unfamiliarity with the task.	× 17
Time shortage.	× 11
Poor human system interface.	× 8
Misperception of risk.	× 4
Inexperience — not lack of training.	× 3
Poor procedures.	× 3
Disturbed sleep patterns.	× 1.6
Monotony and boredom.	× 1.1

outcomes can include anything from the intervention not going quite to plan, to an unfortunate admission to hospital that could have been averted if the resources had been available, to a threat of an assault, etc. It is very important to review clinical practice, and that includes clinical risk management, at every opportunity and not only when the worst outcomes occur. This process should include:

- personal structured reflection
- team reviews
- sentinel event reviews
- external reviews
- coroner's reviews.

Reviewing difficult cases where there were good outcomes will also improve risk management.

Personal structured reflection and review

It is difficult not to include the concept of blame, either of oneself or others, when reviewing a poor outcome. For practice to be reviewed effectively and objectively, the reviewing process should occur as far as possible in a confidential setting, where clinicians can be supported in exploring the event in detail without fear of recrimination. It is out of this type of process that improvements to clinical practice and changes to systems can occur. Team and clinical leaders should have these processes ready to go at all times, but clinicians should also be structuring this work into their everyday practice.

For example, when working in a crisis situation, after the problem has been resolved, it is good practice to spend a moment or two with your colleagues reviewing how it all went. Ask each other if your communication was good, if you would have done things differently at different stages, and if you would do it differently next time, etc. This creates better working relationships, improves communication and is a marvellous opportunity for reflection whilst the event is still fresh. If working on one's own, utilising John's model for structured reflection[6]

BOX 17.1 ANALYSING ADVERSE OUTCOMES

Practice points
- If resource shortfalls hinder a clinician's practice, these should be documented in the file and the team leader should also be informed, preferably in writing.
- Regular auditing, looking for themes of recurring incidents, and feedback to staff helps reduce errors.

1 Description of experience
- What is the 'here and now' experience?
- What essential factors contributed to this experience?
- What were the significant background factors to this experience?

2 Reflection
- What was I trying to achieve?
- Why did I act the way I did?
- What were the consequences of my actions for: myself, patients and colleagues?
- How did I feel about this experience when it was happening?
- Why did I feel that way?
- How did the patients and colleagues feel about it?
- Why did I think they felt that way?
- How did I know this?

3 Alternative actions
- What other choices did I have?
- What would have been the consequences of those other choices?

4 Learning
- How do I now feel about this experience?
- How could I have been more effective?
- What could I do now if faced with a similar situation?
- What have I learned from this experience?

Figure 17.2 **Model for structured reflection**

provides a template to follow. It is brief and easily applied and allows an exploration of the conflict and contradictions between what is practised and what is desirable. Figure 17.2 is an adaptation of the model which can easily be adjusted for group settings after critical incidents.

Implementing change in both practice and systems after a reflective review based on this model is made easier as any change is based on understanding and not simply on emotion generated by the incident.

Team reviews

If the adverse outcome is one which does not require to be reported as a sentinel event, it should not simply be ignored but should be reviewed within the multidisciplinary team. Each team will have its own review process that they have decided upon. As described above, some teams choose to use John's[7] model adapted for group processes. These discussions should be carefully facilitated and the environment should be free of blame and supportive but as far as possible should explore the processes that lead to the adverse outcome. Figure 17.3 expands on the process of structured reflection and takes the review process into an analysis of systems issues.

Who?
- Was involved?
- Was injured?
- Saw the event?
- Has information on events or clinical status of patient prior to the event?

What?
- Was the injured person doing?
- Previous similar events have occurred?
- Action has been taken to prevent recurrence?
- Policies, procedures or guidelines are in place?
- Policies or guidelines were or were not followed?
- Information and/or instruction and/or training and/or supervision was given?
- Were the contributory causes of the event?
- Communication system was in use?

How?
- Could the event have been avoided?
- Could the injury have been avoided?
- Could revision of the treatment plan help?

Why?
- Did the event happen?
- Did the injury occur?
- Did communication fail?
- Was training and/or education not given?
- Were the unsafe conditions permitted?
- Were specific safety and/or treatment instructions not given?
- Was the injured and/or harmed party where they were?

When?
- Did the event occur?
- Was something observed to be wrong?
- Was the person in charge notified?

Where?
- Did the event occur?
- Did the damage occur?
- Were the witnesses at the time?

Figure 17.3 Structured reflection and an analysis of systems issues

Service review, sentinel events and external reviews

Services will have different definitions of what a sentinel event is. Some services divide sentinel events into categories A, B and C. After a serious event, there is usually a requirement for services to review what happened, to learn from the experience and to mitigate future risk. Through these reviews, system and processes, improvements can occur. Dependent on the nature of the event and also on other factors, such as breach of professional codes, external reviews may occur.

Clinicians working in a mental health service should make themselves aware of the reporting requirements and review processes and policies.

As soon as practicable after an adverse event, a meeting should be called to determine ongoing service provision and to consider any management issues which may need to be addressed. These will usually include:

- consideration of whether employees need time off, and the time needed for interviews and planning for return to work
- ongoing service delivery impacts — becoming aware of a service moving into crisis, security needs and the impact of attention by the media.

There should also be a 'staff support — traumatic incident' policy where the following interventions are available:

- Defusing — this may be a simple process of supporting staff whilst they talk about the events of the day before they go home.
- Formal psychological debriefing — although debriefing should be made available, it should be considered with some caution as there are concerns in the literature that this may not be of benefit and, for some clinicians, may cause harm through a process of re-traumatisation.
- Offers of other support services for clinicians. This may include an Employee Assistance Program (EAP) which includes critical incident debriefing and emergency access out of normal hours. Staff may be offered other supports, such as a psychologist on site to drop in and talk to, senior management making themselves available, legal counsel and other additional support options, such as chaplains, etc.

Clinicians will also need to be informed of the review process, who the review team is, and they will need to be informed that they can involve their respective indemnity insurers, union representatives and support person(s).

It is usual nowadays for the report from any review process to be made available to the patient/family and clinicians need to be informed of this.

Being involved in an internal or external review is not an easy process for any clinician. However, in a career working in mental health services, it is likely that this will be an experience which few clinicians will escape. Having some knowledge of the interview process and techniques can be comforting and reassuring. Below are some of the usual interview guidelines for the interviewer.

- Make no attempt to blame or find fault — a key skill at interview is to maintain an open mind and listen to the facts, then draw conclusions.
- Welcome and introduce the interviewee and support person to all interviewers.
- Advise staff to be interviewed of:
  - the purpose of the interview and intent of policy, and that the report will not identify staff
  - their right to have a support person present
  - the terms of reference and offer a copy of the policy
  - how the interview will proceed, including questions and notes
  - expected timeframes, including their opportunity to comment on the draft
  - the involvement of the patient and/or family in the review
  - the outcome of the final report including provision to patient and/or family, coroner and professional bodies, if relevant
  - the fact that any professional or performance issue will not be managed by the review and will be referred to the relevant manager for follow-up.
- Ask the interviewee if they have any questions before commencing the interview.
- Use a comfortable place to ensure the ease of the interviewee.
- Ask for the interviewee's version of what happened. Only ask necessary questions.
- Avoid leading questions. Concentrate on facts not theory.
- Repeat the interviewee's account as you (the interviewer) understand it.
- The interviewee may be emotional. Be empathic and reassuring; remind them:
  - that the purpose of the review is to increase safety and reduce risk, not affix blame
  - that safety can only be increased with their help in identifying all the factors
- Close the interview on a positive note. Check for any further questions.
- Thank the interviewee and support person.

After an interview it is usual for a draft report to be released which should be read carefully for any factual errors.

These types of reviews increasingly take place in an environment of *open disclosure*. Open disclosure is a transparent approach to responding to an incident and/or adverse event that places the patient central to the response. This includes the process of open discussion and ongoing communication with the patient and their support person(s). An open disclosure approach also includes support staff and the development of an open disclosure culture where staff are confident that the associated investigations will have a quality improvement rather than a punitive focus.

After a death

The literature focuses mostly on the care and management of families subsequent to a suicide. However, the same general principles apply to other adverse outcomes. In recent times the practice of supporting the bereaved families of patients has become less common, possibly as a result of the fear of litigation. Avoiding survivors' feelings of abandonment is an integral component of good clinical care and is also desirable, as further family suicides may follow the initial suicide. As well as being good practice, the offering of condolences, saying sorry and being supportive can substantially reduce the risk of further complaints. Saying sorry does not mean accepting blame. 'Stonewalling' many increase anger and grief.[8] For bereaved family members to experience health practitioners as not caring after the death of a loved one tends to create an assumption that the health practitioner did not care to begin with. The provision of outreach to bereaved families is not only humane, but may be the best preventative measure against future complaints.[9]

The mental health worker should contact the family as soon as possible, preferably in person.[10] The aim is to promote effective grieving, bearing in mind displacement of anger and other issues. Some families of patients who have committed suicide display hostility and the mental health worker needs to prepare for this. Open discussion in a private setting should allow the family to ask questions. Mental health workers need to remember that confidentiality continues beyond death.

Many mental health workers will not have been in this situation and, where possible, should be accompanied by a colleague with some experience of this work or with another worker who was involved with the patient.

The importance of continuing to document interventions even after a patient's death should not be forgotten. This is still clinical work which needs to be recorded and communicated.

BOX 17.2 AFTER THE EVENT

Practice points
- Good risk management will not prevent all adverse outcomes.
- Follow-up with family and friends after an adverse outcome is good clinical practice.
- If anxious, take a colleague with you.

Notes

1 Reason J, Mycielska K 1982 *Absent-minded? The Psychology of Mental Lapses and Everyday Errors*. Prentice-Hall, Englewood Cliffs, NJ.

2 Adapted from:Vincent C, Taylor Adams S, Stanhope N 1998 Framework for analysing risk and safety in clinical medicine. *British Medical Journal*, 316:1154–7.

3 Johns C 1995 Achieving effective work as a professional activity. In: Schober JE, Hinchliff SM (eds) *Towards Advanced Nursing Practice*, Arnold, London.

4 Rolfe G, Freshwater D, Jasper M 2001 *Critical Reflection for Nursing and the Helping Professions*. Palgrave Macmillan, Hampshire, UK.

5 Adapted from Williams J, 1988 A database method for assessing and reducing human error to improve operational performance. In: Hagen W (ed.) *ILEEE Fourth Conference on Human Factors and Power Plants*, Institute for Electrical and Electronic Engineers, New York, pp 200–31.

6 Johns, above, n 3.

7 Johns, above, n 3.

8 Litman RE 1982 Hospital suicide: lawsuits and standards. *Suicide and Life Threatening Behaviour*, 12:212–20.

9 Rachlin S 1984 Double jeopardy: suicide and malpractice. *General Hospital Psychiatry*, 6:302–7.

10 Kaye NS, Soreff SM 1991 The psychiatrist's role, responses and responsibilities when a patient commits suicide. *American Journal of Psychiatry*, 148:739–43.

18 Using standardised tools

Despite the current lack of a standardised rating scale that can be used on a regular basis by a general mental health clinician for a wide variety of presentations, it would be remiss not to recognise that the rating scales that are available are of immense use and importance in many areas of mental health work. Furthermore, as understanding of risk factors for specific risks has been increased and refined, the development of standardised rating scales has advanced. Within a forensic environment, standardised rating scales are used extensively.

The use of standardised rating scales on an inpatient ward is perhaps the area where the interface between standardised scales and clinical practice is moving most rapidly. It is an exciting area and will help clinicians become less fearful of incorporating structured approaches into their everyday work.

Standardised rating scales were initially developed within forensic environments to provide a highly structured format to facilitate the assessment of violence. These scales raise an 'index of suspicion' of risk whilst clinical skills allow the context and other factors to be incorporated into a meaningful formulation. Standardised rating scales are the means for assessing which risk factors have relevance for particular risks and have applications in both research and everyday clinical life. 'They enable the clear articulation of the basis for specific estimates of future risk and can clarify sources of disagreement where these occur.'[1] These scales can form an important part of risk management processes when used in conjunction with clinical assessment, although there are disadvantages (as described on page 63). Standardised rating scales draw on research evidence of factors known to be associated with the identified risk. Note should be made once more of the limited usefulness in everyday clinical practice of standardised rating scales that do not include dynamic factors. Scales that limit themselves to static risk factors are of some use in prediction of risk at a population level but have limited place in care of individual patients.

For the general mental health clinician:

> … the initial risk assessment exercise should consist of a structured process of more or less standard questions aimed at eliciting factors increasing the risk (and which will reflect the evidence base around the risk) and which assists clinical judgment. It could be called an *aide-memoire* or a framework. After the clinician addresses these standard questions, it will be possible to determine whether a more in-depth assessment is needed using existing, evidenced-based toolkits for the particular population.[2]

There is no one toolkit which fits all patients and covers all risks. A list of toolkits can be found in Appendix 1 of the UK Department of Health document entitled 'Best Practice in Managing Risk' (2007).[3] New toolkits have been published, including the 'Forensicare Risk Assessment and Management Exercise' (FRAME),[4] in an attempt to incorporate a standardised tool into case management and psychiatric treatment. As yet, for the risks of suicide and self-harm, there is no instrument with a sufficiently strong evidence base.[5] However, Bouch and Marshall (2005) have suggested a useful tool which is worth considering.[6] The most commonly used scale for the assessment of risk of violence on which several of the newer scales are based — the HCR-20[7] — was published in 1997 and has been widely used throughout Canada, America, Europe and Australasia. It is included here (Figure 18.1) to give an idea of what a scale looks like. Within a forensic setting, there is value to be had from applying the HCR-20 at various stages during a patient's treatment as the clinical and risk scores can alter substantially during treatment. Each item is coded on a three-point scale ('absent', 'possibly present' or 'definitely present'). Most of the items in the HCR-20 have been included in the list of risk factors for violence (Table 9.2, page 84–85). Many of them are also included as prompts in the risk form used throughout this book.

To apply the HCR-20 requires prior training, but when used regularly it can be a useful tool to help plan further treatment. The HCR-20 is useful in forensic psychiatry but is much less suitable for general adult psychiatry and is unsuitable for the risk posed by children or by adults with intellectual disabilities.[8]

Using standardised scales to predict violence in inpatient settings

Although standardised scales were developed to predict violence in the longer term, interest has focussed recently on predicting violence in inpatient settings. Several studies have looked at the accuracy of violence predictions on inpatient units. Research has looked at using scales at the time of admission and easily repeated scales during admission. This

HCR-20 risk assessment scheme — items

Historical scale	Factors
H1	Previous violence
H2	Young age at first violent incident
H3	Relationship instability
H4	Employment problems
H5	Substance used problems
H6	Major mental illness
H7	Psychopathy
H8	Early maladjustment
H9	Personality disorder
H10	Prior supervision failure

Clinical scale	
C1	Lack of insight
C2	Negative attitudes
C3	Active symptoms of major mental illness
C4	Impulsivity
C5	Unresponsive to treatment

Risk management scale	
R1	Plans lack feasibility
R2	Exposure to de-stabilisers
R3	Lack of personal support
R4	Non-compliance with the remediation attempts
R5	Stress

(Source: Webster CD, Douglas KS, Eaves D, Hart SD 1997 *HCR-20 Assessing Risk for Violence* (version 2). Mental Health, Law and Policy Institute, Simon Fraser University, Vancouver)

Figure 18.1 Scale for the assessment of risk of violence

work is helping move the use of rating scales away from the time-consuming operations previously required towards simpler scales that are able to be used by all clinicians with little training needed.

One study[9] found that violence on an inpatient ward was best predicted by:

• violence in the week preceding hospitalisation
• general psychopathology score on the Positive and Negative Syndrome Scale[10]
• poor insight into psychotic symptoms.

The last item was the best single predictor. By creating an actuarial prediction model, the researchers were able to correctly identify whether 84% of their sample would exhibit violence during the hospitalisation with a positive predictive power of 80%. This could be used as a simple check at the time of admission.

Another more recent study[11] utilised another quickly applied scale; the Broset Violence Checklist (BVC-CH). This rates six patient behaviours — confusion, irritability, boisterousness, verbal threats, physical threats and attacks on objects — combined with a subjective visual analogue scale. They reported a substantially reduced rate of violence over the 45 913 hospitalisation days studied.

Another scale studied is the Dynamic Appraisal of Situational Aggression (DASA:IV)[12] which includes both dynamic and situational factors.

The DASA:IV assesses the following items:

- negative attitudes
- impulsivity
- irritability
- verbal threats
- sensitivity to perceived provocation
- easily angered when requests are denied
- unwillingness to follow directions.

This can be used to assess risk of imminent aggression on a day-to-day basis.[13] These three studies are important not just because of the usefulness of the rating scale, but also because they promote a climate of risk assessment and management in an environment where violence is not uncommon.

BOX 18.1 STANDARDISED RATING SCALES

Practice points
- Help identify risk factors of relevance for specific risks.
- Can be used in inpatient settings to review risk of violence.
- Are more commonly used in forensic settings.
- Generate the risk factors to be used in structured clinical assessments of risk.
- When used serially, can be an effective measure of change in level of risk.
- Usually require training to be able to administer them.

Further reading on inpatient rating scales

Daffern M 2007 The predictive validity and practical utility of structured schemes used to assess risk for aggression in psychiatric inpatient settings. *Aggression and Violent Behaviour*, 12:116–30.

Doyle M, Dolan M 2006 Predicting community violence from patients discharged from mental health services. *British Journal of Psychiatry*, 189:520–6.

Notes

1 Carroll A 2007 Are violence risk assessment tools clinically useful? *Australian and New Zealand Journal of Psychiatry*, 41:301–7.

2 Royal College of Psychiatrists 2008 Rethinking Risk to Others in Mental Health Services. Final report of a scoping group. Royal College of Psychiatrists College Report CR 150, June.

3 Department of Health 2007 Best Practice in Managing Risk. Principles and Evidence for Best Practice in the Assessment and Management of Risk to Self and Others in Mental Health Services. Document prepared for the National Mental Health Risk Management Programme. Department of Health, London.

4 Carroll A 2008 Risk assessment and management in practice: the Forensicare Risk Assessment and Management Exercise. *Australasian Psychiatry*, 16(6):412–17.

5 Department of Health, above, n 3.

6 Bouch J, Marshall JJ 2005 Suicide risk: structured professional judgment. *Advances in Psychiatric Treatment*, 11:84–91.

7 Webster CD, Douglas KS, Eaves D, Hart SD 1997 *HCR-20 Assessing Risk for Violence* (version 2). Mental Health, Law and Policy Institute, Simon Fraser University, Vancouver.

8 Royal College of Psychiatrists, above, n 2.

9 Arango C, Barba AC, Gonzalez-Salvador T, Ordonez AC 1999 Violence in inpatients with schizophrenia; a prospective study. *Schizophrenia Bulletin*, 25:493–503.

10 The PANSS, or the Positive and Negative Syndrome Scale, is a rating scale used for measuring symptom severity of patients with schizophrenia.

11 Abderhalden C, Needham I, Halfens R, Haug H, Fischer JE 2008 Structured risk assessment and violence in acute psychiatric wards: randomised controlled trial. *British Journal of Psychiatry*, 193:44–50.

12 Ogloff JRP, Daffern M 2003 *The Assessment of Inpatient Aggression at the Thomas Embling Hospital: Towards the Dynamic Appraisal of Inpatient Aggression*. Forensicare, Victorian Institute of Forensic Mental Health Fourth Annual Research Report to Council, 1 July 2002–30 June 2003.

13 Barry-Walsh J, Daffern M, Duncan S, Ogloff J 2009 The prediction of imminent aggression in patients with mental illness and/or intellectual disability using the Dynamic Appraisal of Situational Aggression instrument. *Australian Psychiatry*, vol 17 no 6.

APPENDICES

Appendix 1
Formats for documenting risk
Risk management plan

RISK ASSESSMENT AND MANAGEMENT FORM	
DATE OF PLAN	**NAME OF PATIENT** Place label here
EXPIRY DATE (maximum – 6 months)	Surname: Given name: DOB: Patient number:

CURRENT DIAGNOSES AND CLINICAL CONCERNS
Include personality traits/disorder.

CURRENT RISKS
What is/are the risk/s? Who is the risk to, what means might be used and where might it happen?

PREVIOUS EPISODES OF THE RISK(S) Where did it happen, to whom and when? What was the context — illness, situational factors, substance use, not taking medications? Document each episode in as much detail as possible. Identify <u>recurring patterns (risk scenarios)</u> from this information.

WHAT ARE THE FUNCTIONS OF THE RISK BEHAVIOURS? For example, acting on delusions or hallucinations, self-harm reducing tension or distress, violence or threats being effective, etc.	**WHAT INTERVENTIONS HELP ADDRESS THESE FACTORS? WHAT SKILLS ARE BEING DEVELOPED TO DO THIS?** For example, reality orientation, self-soothing, cognitive skills, dialectical behaviour therapy (DBT) skills, etc.

WHAT IN THIS PERSON'S HISTORY CONTRIBUTES TO INCREASING RISK?
For example, history of substance use, conduct disorder, impulsivity, etc. Use the validated scales from your training manual

WHAT MENTAL STATE FACTORS INCREASE THESE RISKS? For example, hallucinations, delusions, feelings of rejection, depression, etc.	**WHAT INTERVENTIONS HELP ADDRESS THESE FACTORS?** For example, compliance with medication, reduced stress.
Identify early warning signs and triggers of these factors. Who notices the changes first?	
WHAT EXTERNAL, ENVIRONMENTAL OR SITUATIONAL FACTORS AFFECT THE RISK? For example, substance use, living conditions, relationship problems, not taking medication, etc.	**WHAT INTERVENTIONS HELP ADDRESS THESE FACTORS?** For example, respite, reducing drug use, phoning a friend.
WHAT SKILLS OR RESOURCES ARE THE PROTECTIVE FACTORS? For example, insight into illness, supportive family, stable accommodation, compliance with medication, etc.	**WHO ELSE IS INVOLVED IN THE CARE AND TREATMENT OF THIS PATIENT?** For example, family, friends, etc.

TEAMS AND CLINICIANS INVOLVED

THIS FORM MUST INCLUDE A FACE SHEET and TREATMENT PLAN

COMPULSORY COPY TO: Crisis Team
ALSO COPIED TO: ☐ Patient ☐ Family ☐ GP ☐ Emergency Department
☐ Accommodation provider ☐ Other (specify)

PRINT NAME AND DESIGNATION	**Date**	**Time**

Have you put enough information in this form to help a colleague treat and care for this patient in an emergency?

Treatment plan with prompts for management of risk

Treatment Plan and Review		
Date of plan:	**NAME OF PATIENT**	Place label here
Date of expiry of plan:(maximum — 6 months)	Surname: DOB:	Given name: NHI:
Current clinical concerns. Current diagnoses and co-existing disorders.		
Short-term treatment goals. Consider medical, psychological, social, pharmacological goals.	**What interventions are planned to achieve the goals?**	
Longer-term treatment goals. Consider medical, psychological, social, pharmacological goals, etc	**What interventions are planned to achieve the goals?**	
Early warning signs and triggers for relapse.	**Strategies, supports and Interventions.**	
Relapse indicators	**Strategies, supports and interventions**	

Team and clinicians involved

- **Does the patient need a risk management plan? Does this plan address the management of the risk factors?**
- **Does the current plan need updating?**
- Treatment plan copied to:

☐ Crisis Team ☐ Patient ☐ Family ☐ GP ☐ Emergency Department
☐ Other (specify)

Clinician signature:	Date:
Print name and designation:	
Patient signature:	Time:

TREATMENT REVIEW (within 6 months of the plan being made). After this review, a new treatment plan should be generated.

Signed   Date

Triage form with prompts for risk

Triage Form	
Date:	**NAME OF PATIENT** Place label here Surname: Given name: DOB: NHI:

Type of contact. For example, *telephone, face to face. Who is making the contact?*

Nature of the contact. *What is the problem? What happened? Seriousness of the event? Effect of event on the patient? Change to mental state? What is the patient requesting?*

Risk issues. *Risk to self and/or others? Do you need to complete a risk management plan?*

Outcome and action taken. *Short-term goals and interventions suggested.*

Team and clinicians involved:

Triage form copied to: (attach cover sheet)

☐ Crisis Team   ☐ Patient   ☐ Family   ☐ GP   ☐ Emergency Department
☐ Accommodation Provider   ☐ Other (specify)

Clinician signature:	Date:
Print name and designation:	Time:

Appendix 2
Teaching risk assessment and management

Teaching clinical risk assessment and management to mental health practitioners is seen as being a core requirement for most mental health services. In some countries it is compulsory for all clinicians to be trained in risk every 3 years. For most junior practitioners, it would be inappropriate to be trained in utilising standardised rating scales without first having a reasonable grounding in basic theory, assessment and management skills.

In my current mental health service, and in the surrounding regions, a small group of trainers has now taught many clinicians on risk assessment and management. Over a period of 5 years, the training has been modified extensively. We have found that sending out background reading on basic concepts and theory prior to a workshop is advantageous. Even if some participants do not avail themselves of the background reading, most do and they bring some knowledge and interest into their training.

The training is usually a 1 day workshop — we found that a half day workshop is too short to adequately ground clinicians in the clinical skills which they need. The process of the day is firstly a brief recap of the background reading (part one of the current book) followed by clinical examples of three or four cases which are used during the rest of the day to serve as the basis for learning about assessment, management, documentation and communication.

The cases are varied dependent on the group attending the workshop, but usually include one case of violence, one case of suicidality and another of chronic suicidality. For child and family services the cases are rewritten for their age group and similarly for psychogeriatric services. There is also a set of cases written for practitioners from intellectual disability services.

We have found that it is best to write the cases in such a way that there will be a degree of uncertainty about optimal management for the patients. For example, the case of a violent patient is written in such a way that there may be discussion generated about whether confidentiality should be breached or whether the patient should be compulsorily detained. For the suicidal patient, there will be uncertainty about whether the patient should be admitted to hospital or not.

As clinical risk assessment and management is best undertaken with a colleague or within the multidisciplinary team, the work of the day is predominantly done either in small groups or in the large team group. The preferable maximum number of participants is approximately 25.

We focus a lot on the quality of the documentation and emphasise repeatedly that the documentation should be written in such a way that a colleague looking after a patient on a different shift should be able to quickly familiarise themselves with the patient's risks. Passing around completed documentation from one group to another at an early stage in the workshop usually leads to a rapid improvement in the quality of documentation. The groups are mixed up after each of the cases.

At some stage during the day it is hoped that there will be sufficient discussion within the group to enable a risk/benefit analysis to be undertaken. The cases should be written in such a way that this is likely to happen. The cases should be written so that there is a maximum of discussion within the group, which should be facilitated by the presenters. There should be no set answers for any of the cases and the essence of the day is to teach skills. Frequently, there are complaints that not enough clinical information has been included in the case examples. This should be acknowledged early on and we suggest that clinicians use their creativity in imagining what else might have been happening in the scenario and utilising that information when documenting their findings.

We have found that training individual teams works best. Follow-up about 3 weeks later with a visit to the team, offering support for individual clinicians working in risk management, helps reinforce the training.

Appendix 3
Exercises — answers and discussions

The 'answers' given in the exercises may well differ from yours in regard to the clinical decisions made. If your answers vary widely from those given here, ask a colleague for their thoughts. This is common in clinical practice and it is a useful reminder to confer with your colleagues if you have doubt. Many of the scenarios have limited clinical information which you may find frustrating. It is impossible to generate scenarios which have all the information that you would glean from routine work. What will be missing especially will be the non-verbal information which is a vital part of any patient interaction. Use the scenarios as exercises only, accepting that some information that you would like to have will be lacking. Where you are asked to fill in areas for which information has not been given, be creative and use your clinical judgment. The exercises are to get you used to the processes of risk assessment, management and documentation and have no right or wrong answers.

Chapter 3

1 Tonight there is a high likelihood of Richard committing suicide if he is left alone. He has the means (a knife) and believes that his family would be better off without him (likely a depressive cognition). However, he is already being seen by a mental health service and he is unlikely to be left on his own tonight, which will lower the risk substantially.

2 The likelihood is now much lower as he is in a contained environment in which he can be observed and monitored closely. The context is very different. The change from being in the community to the secure environment of an inpatient psychiatric unit can change the likelihood of risk substantially.

3 The likelihood of Richard committing suicide is now low. The internal and situational dynamic factors have changed. The situational factors will change again when Richard is discharged and the likelihood of suicide may increase again for a while. The nature of the risk has not changed throughout his illness: it remains suicide.

Chapter 7
Exercise 1 — level of risk changing over time

Consideration of your own risk thermostat should be routine. It should occur with every patient interaction! Does your heart go out to Alison and her family or are you tired as you've been working for 12 hours?

Are you anxious about the bed state and will this affect your decision-making? Are you worried about the media getting the story if you don't admit Alison and she kills herself?

The people involved in the system caring for Alison are the community mental health team, her supportive family and probably the hospital inpatient unit. Other systemic components are the resource restrictions of limited beds. If she is not admitted to hospital, you will be using the wider resources of the mental health services in the form of crisis respite, home-based treatment etc. Finally, there will be an implication for the care of other patients if Alison is admitted to hospital and takes the last bed. If you are fearful of media coverage, consider discussing this with a senior colleague to determine the best approach to take.

Chapter 9
Exercise 1 — Monique

> **CURRENT DIAGNOSES AND CLINICAL CONCERNS** *Include personality traits/disorder.*
>
> Monique suffers from schizophrenia. The current difficulty is that her boyfriend has left her and she is distraught.
>
> **CURRENT RISKS** *What is/are the risk/s? Who is the risk is to, what means might be used and where might it happen?*
>
> Staff in the supported accommodation hostel are fearful that Monique is at risk of suicide. She may also be at risk of relapsing back into her psychosis or develop a depressive episode. Given the loss of her relationship, the next few weeks are going to be more critical. At this stage there is insufficient information to know what means Monique is thinking about using if she is suicidal.

Exercise 2 — Phoebe

> **CURRENT DIAGNOSES AND CLINICAL CONCERNS** *Include personality traits/disorder.*
>
> Phoebe is an 83-year-old woman with a major depressive disorder. She has not eaten for 3 days.
>
> **CURRENT RISKS** *What is/are the risk to, what means might be used and where might it happen?*
>
> Phoebe is at high risk of dying within the next 24 hours from dehydration. There will be a risk of suicide because she is suffering from a depressive illness but this appears to be a much lower risk than the risk of death from dehydration. It is more likely that she will die from self-neglect rather than using any particular means to kill herself.

Exercise 3 — Colin

CURRENT DIAGNOSES AND CLINICAL CONCERNS *Include personality traits/disorder.*

Colin has just arrived from another city. He is unknown to services. He was picked up by the police for shaking his fist at passers by and chanting.

CURRENT RISKS *What is/are the risk/s? Who is the risk to, what means might be used and where might it happen?*

Colin presents with a risk of being violent. At this stage it is uncertain what the level of risk is, but he is more likely to use his fists and violence might be directed towards any member of the public. It is unknown whether he has a weapon or if there is a past history of violence.

Exercise 4 — Rebecca

CURRENT DIAGNOSES AND CLINICAL CONCERNS *Include personality traits/disorder.*

Rebecca has borderline personality disorder. She has had an argument with her boyfriend.

CURRENT RISKS *What is/are the risk/s? Who is the risk to, what means might be used and where might it happen?*

Rebecca is at risk of self-harm. Rebecca's illness is characterised by impulsivity and the self-harm is more likely to happen within the next few hours if it occurs at all. She tends to self-harm at home using razor blades that she keeps in her handbag.

Exercise 5 — Monique (continued)

CURRENT DIAGNOSES AND CLINICAL CONCERNS

Monique has schizophrenia characterised by both positive and negative symptoms. Her hallucinations sometimes tell her to hurt herself. Her relationship has just ended. She smokes marijuana occasionally.

CURRENT RISKS

Staff in the supported accommodation hostel where Monique lives are concerned that she may have developed suicidal intent.
She may be at risk of relapse of psychosis.

PREVIOUS EPISODES OF THE RISK(S)

Monique has attempted suicide three times previously, each episode occurring in the context of a relapse of her psychotic illness. She has always overdosed on her medication. Critical risk factors are likely to be episodes of psychosis, especially if her auditory hallucinations tell her to harm herself.

WHAT IN THIS PERSON'S HISTORY CONTRIBUTES TO INCREASING RISK?

Long-term cannabis abuse. Little memory about her childhood. Father has a diagnosis of schizophrenia. Chronic psychotic symptoms. Chronic negative symptoms. Termination of pregnancy and adoption of the baby of subsequent pregnancy.

WHAT MENTAL STATE FACTORS INCREASE THESE RISKS?

Currently Monique is frequently tearful and withdrawn. Staff have a gut feeling that she is suicidal. Sometimes Monique's voices tell her to hurt herself. Her capacity to resist her voices lessens as the voices become more intense.

Identify early warning signs and triggers of these factors. Who notices the changes first?

When Monique's self-cares deteriorate, this is often an early warning sign. She also becomes preoccupied, withdrawn and tearful.

WHAT EXTERNAL, ENVIRONMENTAL OR SITUATIONAL FACTORS AFFECT THE RISK?

Monique's relationship with her boyfriend ended 2 weeks ago and she continues to smoke cannabis from time to time. She has always been vulnerable to abuse by others.

WHAT SKILLS OR RESOURCES ARE THE PROTECTIVE FACTORS?

Monique's mother is supportive. The support staff are clearly concerned about Monique.

Exercise 6 — Colin (continued)

CURRENT DIAGNOSES AND CLINICAL CONCERNS

Colin has a psychotic illness characterised by persecutory delusions and delusions of reference. His use of cannabis seems to make his psychosis worse.

CURRENT RISKS

In the context of a psychotic illness, Colin is currently at risk of assaulting either his flatmate or people on the street as a result of feeling persecuted. It is not known if he has a weapon.

PREVIOUS EPISODES OF THE RISK(S)

Colin has three convictions for assault. These have all occurred in the context of being drunk. Although he says he wouldn't hurt a fly, it is unknown if he has had other episodes of violence when drunk or even when sober.

WHAT IN THIS PERSON'S HISTORY CONTRIBUTES TO INCREASING RISK?

Colin has a long history of smoking cannabis and heavy alcohol use. He has a past history of three convictions for assault all of which occurred when he was drunk. The last episode occurred 13 years ago.

WHAT MENTAL STATE FACTORS INCREASE THESE RISKS?

Colin has a 6-month history of paranoid delusions believing there were recording devices in his room and ideas of reference. These symptoms are continuing although settling slightly. However, he is becoming increasingly angry about what is going on.

Identify early warning signs and triggers of these factors. Who notices the changes first?

If Colin is new to your town, he has probably moved to escape his sense of being persecuted. He tends to wander the streets reciting prayers at these times. He may also check for recording devices when seen for assessment.

WHAT EXTERNAL, ENVIRONMENTAL OR SITUATIONAL FACTORS AFFECT THE RISK?

Until very recently Colin has continued to smoke cannabis. He has recently changed accommodation and, at this time, is reluctant to take medication. He is not currently drinking.

WHAT SKILLS OR RESOURCES ARE THE PROTECTIVE FACTORS?

Colin is developing some insight that cannabis may be problematic. In the last few weeks he decided to stop smoking cannabis and has noticed that his paranoia has settled slightly. He has not been violent for 13 years and, during this current episode of illness, there has been no history of violence. Reciting prayers is protective for Colin as well as being an early warning sign.

Chapter 10

Exercise 1 — Colin (continued)

Management and treatment possibilities	Risk	Benefit
Admit to hospital involuntarily	Admitting Colin involuntarily risks alienating him at the start of his treatment. The environment of the ward may increase the risk of violence.	Further assessment of the risk of violence.
Arrange follow-up sooner than the few weeks that Colin has suggested	Colin may become violent in the community.	The therapeutic alliance with Colin is not damaged and is improved by not imposing treatment. He is treated in the least restrictive environment.
Other management and treatment options*		

* Additional rows such as this may be added depending upon your individual organisation's service options (e.g. a day hospital or a crisis respite bed may be available).

Exercise 2 — Fred

Management and treatment possibilities	Risk	Benefit
Continue with Haldol	Positive symptoms don't change.	No concerns about compliance.
Start clozapine	He may forget to take the medication. Possibility of severe side effects.	His schizophrenia improves and he may enter into remission.

Exercise 3 — Jane

Management and treatment possibilities	Risk	Benefit
Admit to psychiatric unit	She will be away from her supportive family and the strange environment may make her psychosis worse.	Closer assessment of the mental state and opportunity to commence medication with close observation.
Ask if she can stay on the medical ward	Nursing staff here are not trained to observe mental state. Uses precious medical beds.	You get a couple of days for further observation whilst working out what to do.
Send her home with close follow-up by the Community Mental Health Team (CMHT)	The time lag between arriving home and the CMHT follow-up.	She stays in close contact with her family and is treated in the least restrictive environment.
Transfer her to crisis respite and the day hospital	She will be away from her supportive family and the strange environment may make her psychosis worse.	Closer assessment of the mental state and opportunity to commence medication with close observation. Does not use a hospital bed.
Discharge home with follow-up by the home-based treatment team	If her psychosis worsens, she may leave her home precipitously.	She stays with her family and is able to have intensive treatment in the least restrictive environment.

Exercise 4 — Roger

Treatment possibilities	Risk	Benefit
Stay in hospital	Roger may regress and self-harm more frequently. 'Affect storms' (see glossary) increase this risk. He may lose touch with his community supports. At risk of becoming institutionalised.	He is more likely to stay alive.
Treat in the community	Roger may kill himself (albeit accidentally).	Doesn't regress. Can get support from friends more easily. Doesn't lose community supports. Can continue with usual treatment.

Exercise 5 — alcohol and drug example (Gillian)

Treatment possibilities	Risk	Benefit
Discontinue methadone immediately	This may put the unborn baby at risk. Gillian may start taking illicit opiates which further compromise the foetus.	Gillian does not put anybody else at risk.
Daily dispense methadone from clinic	She may not attend daily and choose to use opiates from the street.	The risks of diversion are minimised. We are able to monitor her dose and mental state closely.
Daily dispense methadone from pharmacy	She may divert her methadone.	There are no particular advantages to continuing with the present treatment regimen.
Withdraw from methadone during second trimester	She is on a reasonably high dose of methadone and this would be risky. She is likely to start using illicit opiates.	Gillian would put fewer people at risk.
Maintain on methadone until the end of pregnancy, and then withdraw	She would likely start using illicit opiates again.	The unborn baby is cared for until birth.
Report her to the police for diverting her methadone	This is not an option as we would be breaching confidentiality. (For duty to warn and protect see page X.)	

Chapter 11

Exercise 1 — Depression and post-traumatic stress disorder (PTSD)

This is a difficult example as you have not been given much history. Obviously, you will want to spend more time with David assessing the risk and getting collateral history. In this completed example, extra information has been included for completeness although the information was not given in the history.

CURRENT DIAGNOSES AND CLINICAL CONCERNS

David is a 42-year-old man suffering from a major depressive disorder which has been resistive to usual treatment interventions. More recently, he has developed symptoms of PTSD after being reminded of being abused when younger.

CURRENT RISKS

The primary risk for David is of suicide. Currently, David has not considered what means he might use and there is no active suicidal intent. However, his depressive illness has worsened in recent weeks.
David also has contemplated the idea of vengeance against the perpetrator of the childhood abuse. He has violent feelings but no plans.

PREVIOUS EPISODES OF THE RISK(S)

There is no known history of either suicidal acts or violence.

WHAT ARE THE FUNCTIONS OF THE RISK BEHAVIOUR?

At times, the degree of torment that David experiences from his depression has led him to believe that suicide would be a relief. He also feels that his parents would be devastated if he killed himself.
David has a sense that if justice was served upon the teacher that he would get 'closure' and that his depression would lift immediately. He has said that he would experience remorse if he personally attacked the teacher, although the thought has crossed his mind.

WHAT IN THIS PERSON'S HISTORY CONTRIBUTES TO INCREASING RISK?

David does not use alcohol or drugs. There is no history of impulsivity or personality disorder.

WHAT MENTAL STATE FACTORS INCREASE THESE RISKS?

The suicide risk is linked to his depressive symptomatology. Currently he is not actively suicidal. He is more likely to be violent during dissociative states. If his depression worsens, he may have a lower threshold for violence.
Identify early warning signs and triggers of these factors. Who notices the changes first?
David may present with increasing tearfulness, increased anger and also with deteriorating sleep patterns.

WHAT EXTERNAL, ENVIRONMENTAL OR SITUATIONAL FACTORS AFFECT THE RISK?

If David were to bump into the man who perpetrated the abuse, the risk of violence would be greater.

WHAT SKILLS OR RESOURCES ARE THE PROTECTIVE FACTORS?	WHO ELSE IS INVOLVED IN THE CARE AND TREATMENT OF THIS PATIENT?
Although David is insightful into his illness, the worsening depression and episodes of dissociation are concerning. Currently the preoccupation with vengeance is a protective factor for suicide.	From the history, David's only support currently is the mental health team.

TEAMS AND CLINICIANS INVOLVED

Case Manager Jo de Bier and Dr James Mc Psyche, Consultant Psychiatrist. South Community Team, St Elsewhere's Health Trust.
Phone 04 488834

Have you put enough information in this form to help a colleague treat and care for this patient in an emergency?

Exercise 2 — child and family example

Discussion

This is an example of a situation where the patient is vulnerable and exposed to risks from others. As you become aware of more of the details of what is happening in the home environment, it would be easy to expand on some of the risk factors. It may well be important to document something about his mother's capacity to cope with stressful situations. The completed form below describes the risk as violence. Some clinicians may find this term too strong and wish to use a milder term. This would be a useful discussion in a multidisciplinary team (MDT) forum.

CURRENT DIAGNOSES AND CLINICAL CONCERNS

Mike suffers from enuresis and school phobia which arose following the separation of his parents.

CURRENT RISKS

Mike is at risk of violence, possibly at the hand of his mother, although this is unclear at the moment. The violence may be evidence of his mother no longer coping well and not knowing how to manage the situation.

PREVIOUS EPISODES OF THE RISK(S)

As yet, no previous episodes of violence have been discovered.

WHAT ARE THE FUNCTIONS OF THE RISK BEHAVIOUR?

Mike's mother has been trying to persuade him to go to school and used excessive physical methods to try and encourage him. There is some concern that she may be getting depressed.

WHAT IN THIS PERSON'S HISTORY CONTRIBUTES TO INCREASING RISK?

The separation of his parents has been an important factor. As yet, no other factors have been recognised.

WHAT MENTAL STATE FACTORS INCREASE THESE RISKS?

His school phobia puts him at risk of violence as he can become stubborn and angry as a way of expressing his fear of going to school.

Identify early warning signs and triggers of these factors. Who notices the changes first?
Monday mornings may be a vulnerable time.

WHAT EXTERNAL, ENVIRONMENTAL OR SITUATIONAL FACTORS AFFECT THE RISK?

He is more vulnerable when he is staying with his mother. The trauma of his parents' separation has not been resolved for Mike.

WHAT SKILLS OR RESOURCES ARE THE PROTECTIVE FACTORS?	WHO ELSE IS INVOLVED IN THE CARE AND TREATMENT OF THIS PATIENT?
The family are well engaged in treatment with Child and Adolescent Services. His mother is very keen to learn other techniques to help Mike attend school.	Mike is cared for predominantly by his mother and has each weekend with his father. His paternal grandparents are closely involved.

Have you put enough information in this form to help a colleague treat and care for this patient in an emergency?

Exercise 3 — an example of using the model for exploring relapse prevention

Discussion

Brian does not really have any substantive risks such as violence or suicide. One could imagine that his 'verbal aggressiveness' could lead to violence. The value of completing a risk plan in this instance is that it highlights some of the early warning signs, relapse indicators and triggers which may be of relevance. The fact that his wife picks up the early warning signs of a relapse first is always going to be important. An exploration of how she 'knows' he is getting ill will need to be undertaken. If your treatment plan documentation also includes exploration of early warning signs, triggers and relapse indicators, it may not be necessary to fill out a risk plan. As mentioned in Chapter 8, if you are not sure whether you should be filling out a risk plan, it is always easy to complete the plan if the risk is minimal and there will have been little time wasted. As can be seen from the documentation below, the risk is minimal and the form was very quick to complete. However there is useful information about risks of relapse and early warning signs which can be quickly 'cut and pasted' into the treatment plan.

CURRENT DIAGNOSES AND CLINICAL CONCERNS
Brian suffers from schizoaffective disorder characterised by manic episodes and persecutory ideation. His compliance with medication is variable.

CURRENT RISKS
When manic, Brian becomes disinhibited, reckless and impulsive. During his last episode of illness, he stole a racehorse and rode it bareback to his home.

PREVIOUS EPISODES OF THE RISK(S)
There is no history of violence but he can be verbally aggressive. No other risks noted. An early warning sign might be poor compliance with medication.

WHAT ARE THE FUNCTIONS OF THE RISK BEHAVIOUR?
When ill, Brian usually says that he is having the time of his life and he is loath to accept treatment. When well, he is increasingly aware of the effects that his illness is having on his life.

WHAT IN THIS PERSON'S HISTORY CONTRIBUTES TO INCREASING RISK?
Nil known.

WHAT MENTAL STATE FACTORS INCREASE THESE RISKS?
Brian's manic symptoms make him more impulsive and reckless. His psychotic symptoms seem to make him more verbally aggressive.
Identify early warning signs and triggers of these factors. Who notices the changes first?   Brian usually presents with poor sleep as the first indication of a relapse. His wife invariably notices changes in his mental state first.

WHAT EXTERNAL, ENVIRONMENTAL OR SITUATIONAL FACTORS AFFECT THE RISK?
Brian's compliance with medication is partial and puts him at risk of relapse.

WHAT SKILLS OR RESOURCES ARE THE PROTECTIVE FACTORS?	WHO ELSE IS INVOLVED IN THE CARE AND TREATMENT OF THIS PATIENT?
Although Brian does not take his medication all the time, he does take it reasonably often.	Brian is well supported by his wife and he has known his case manager for some years.

Have you put enough information in this form to help a colleague treat and care for this patient in an emergency?

Exercise 4 — alcohol and drug example

Discussion

As in the previous example, the risks are not of violence or suicide but are the common risk seen in alcohol and drug services of the patient continuing to drive. This problem may lead you to look up your local guidelines about patients continuing to drive and your responsibilities to inform the local vehicle licensing agency. As in the previous example, completing this form, which is quite quick, also throws up factors which need to be addressed in the treatment plan. A common problem in alcohol and drug services is use of the substance making the psychiatric problem worse, and vice versa.

CURRENT DIAGNOSES AND CLINICAL CONCERNS

Rachel is alcohol dependent and has been self-medicating to manage her generalised anxiety disorder and panic. It is quite likely that the alcohol abuse perpetuates her anxiety disorder. There is a possibility that she suffers from post-traumatic stress disorder but this has not been verified as yet. Her marriage is currently stressed.

CURRENT RISKS

Rachel's biggest risk is of some form of motor vehicle accident as a result of driving whilst inebriated. This may involve just Rachel but she is also putting her children and other road users at risk. Rachel's marriage is also at risk. Rachel is also at risk of other accidents whilst inebriated.

PREVIOUS EPISODES OF THE RISK(S)

Four months ago Rachel had a motor vehicle accident whilst inebriated. Around the same time, she also fell down the stairs.
Any use of alcohol should be seen as an early warning sign. Triggers for alcohol use include her anxiety disorder and memories of the previous date rape.

WHAT ARE THE FUNCTIONS OF THE RISK BEHAVIOUR?

Rachel's alcoholism is reinforcing in that it allows her to avoid addressing her other difficulties and also allows her to forget.

WHAT IN THIS PERSON'S HISTORY CONTRIBUTES TO INCREASING RISK?

Her alcoholism is the biggest historic risk factor. The date rape is also likely to be of substantial relevance although this has not been fully explored as yet. Rachel says that she has put it behind her but this currently seems unlikely.

WHAT MENTAL STATE FACTORS INCREASE THESE RISKS?

Rachel will always be most at risk when inebriated. When sober, she is always remorseful for her behaviour but this is insufficient to reduce the risk. Her anxiety and panic make it more likely that she will drink.

Identify early warning signs and triggers of these factors. Who notices the changes first?
Rachel's husband notices when Rachel is slipping before she does but she usually disagrees with his concern.

WHAT EXTERNAL, ENVIRONMENTAL OR SITUATIONAL FACTORS AFFECT THE RISK?
Rachel's marital disharmony perpetuates her drinking although she does not feel ready to enter into couple counselling. Her husband is unaware of her feelings.

WHAT SKILLS OR RESOURCES ARE THE PROTECTIVE FACTORS?	**WHO ELSE IS INVOLVED IN THE CARE AND TREATMENT OF THIS PATIENT?**
Rachel is engaged in treatment for her substance abuse, still on an outpatient basis. Rachel's marriage is possibly protective.	Rachel has few supports in her life other than her husband.

Have you put enough information in this form to help a colleague treat and care for this patient in an emergency?

Exercise 5 — opioid substitution example

Discussion

This is a common scenario in many opioid substitution clinics. As with several of the other examples, documenting the risks highlights many of the areas which need to be addressed within the treatment plan. This type of presentation has many treatment possibilities which may benefit from a risk/benefit analysis when treatment options are being considered. See the example on page 100.

Note: COP is an abbreviation for 'consume on premises'. Patients taking methadone are often required to consume their medication in the pharmacy under the supervision of the pharmacist.

CURRENT DIAGNOSES AND CLINICAL CONCERNS
Melanie is opioid dependent and has a needle fixation. A new clinical concern currently is that her boyfriend is also opioid dependent and is on the waiting list for substitution treatment.

CURRENT RISKS
Melanie is at risk of physical complications from repeated injections. Her partner Greg is at risk of overdose if Melanie gives him some of her methadone. She is at risk of giving Greg her methadone or being 'stood over' by him.

PREVIOUS EPISODES OF THE RISK(S)
Melanie has a well-documented needle fixation. This has been difficult to manage given the rural setting in which she lives. Any take-aways that she has are likely to be utilised intravenously or given to Greg.

WHAT ARE THE FUNCTIONS OF THE RISK BEHAVIOUR?

Melanie's injecting behaviour is very reinforcing as the pleasure it gives her is much greater than when she takes methadone orally. The risk of physical complications such as abscesses is outweighed by the pleasure she gets from injecting.

Melanie is also likely to share her methadone with her boyfriend who is waiting to go on the program. As well as destabilising Melanie, he will be at risk of overdose.

WHAT IN THIS PERSON'S HISTORY CONTRIBUTES TO INCREASING RISK?

Melanie's injecting behaviour is longstanding and has been difficult to manage because of her living so far away from a pharmacy which is open on Sundays.

WHAT MENTAL STATE FACTORS INCREASE THESE RISKS?

Melanie is vulnerable to Greg standing over her and demanding methadone. Her fear of him leaving her makes it more likely that she will give him some of her methadone.
Identify early warning signs and triggers of these factors. Who notices the changes first?

WHAT EXTERNAL, ENVIRONMENTAL OR SITUATIONAL FACTORS AFFECT THE RISK?

Melanie lives a long way from a pharmacy which is open on Sundays and it is difficult to organise for her to have 7 COPs.

WHAT SKILLS OR RESOURCES ARE THE PROTECTIVE FACTORS?	WHO ELSE IS INVOLVED IN THE CARE AND TREATMENT OF THIS PATIENT?
Melanie is well engaged with the methadone program. If her partner is able to come onto the program quickly, the risks will be reduced substantially. She is hoping to be transferred to suboxone, if this becomes available.	Apart from her good relationship with her case manager, Melanie has no other contacts apart from her partner.

Have you put enough information in this form to help a colleague treat and care for this patient in an emergency?

Chapter 12
Exercise 1 — Colin (continued)

Risk Assessment and Management Form			
DATE OF PLAN	25 June 2010	**NAME OF PATIENT**	Place label here
REVIEW DATE (maximum— 6 months)	25 September 2010	Surname:	Given name: *Colin*
		DOB:	Patient ID number:

CURRENT DIAGNOSES AND CLINICAL CONCERNS
Include personality traits/disorder.

Colin is suffering from a delusional disorder — paranoid type in which he feels that people are watching him. History of personality development is currently unknown.

CURRENT RISKS
What is/are the risk/s? Who is the risk to, what means might be used and where might it happen?

Colin is at risk of being violent. The risk is most likely to be towards anybody whom he perceives as watching or persecuting him. He tends to use his fists rather than any weapon.

PREVIOUS EPISODES OF THE RISK(S) Where did it happen, to whom and when? What was the context — illness, situational factors, substance use, not taking medications? Document each episode in as much detail as possible. Identify recurring patterns (risk scenarios) from this information.

Colin was violent on three occasions in his late teens and early 20s. These all occurred when he was drunk and got into brawls in the pub. It's relevant to note that he was convicted on each occasion. In the past he had a low threshold for using his fists to resolve arguments. **Identify early warning signs and triggers of these factors.**

WHAT ARE THE FUNCTIONS OF THE RISK BEHAVIOURS? For example, acting on delusions or hallucinations; self-harm reducing tension or distress, violence or threats being effective.	**WHAT INTERVENTIONS HELP ADDRESS THESE FACTORS? WHAT SKILLS ARE BEING DEVELOPED TO DO THIS?** For example, reality orientation, self-soothing, cognitive skills, DBT skills, etc.
It is likely that Colin would only become violent if he felt that he needed to protect himself from perceived persecution by others. Violence in the absence of psychosis is unlikely unless he is drunk and gets into an argument although this has become less likely as he gets older.	Colin is beginning to recognise that he doesn't know how else to deal with threats other than using his fists. He has agreed to attend an anger management course starting soon.

WHAT IN THIS PERSON'S HISTORY CONTRIBUTES TO INCREASING RISK?
For example, substance use, conduct disorder, impulsivity etc. Use the validated scales from your training manual.

Colin has had a low threshold for violence in the past, especially in the context of being drunk. He continues to use drugs, including alcohol. The last conviction was 13 years ago, however, and he is currently saying he doesn't want to go to prison.

WHAT MENTAL STATE FACTORS INCREASE THESE RISKS? For example, hallucinations, delusions, feelings of rejection, depression etc.	WHAT INTERVENTIONS HELP ADDRESS THESE FACTORS? For example, compliance with medication, reduced stress, etc.
Colin is most likely to be violent when he is suffering paranoid delusions or ideas of reference: he has felt that people are monitoring him with cameras and at times speaking to him from the television. If he is angry, this is probably a risk factor.	Written by Colin Try to stay off cannabis. Remind myself that this is likely to be my illness and get in touch with my case manager. Make sure I am taking my medication. See my case manager and doctor urgently
Identify early warning signs and triggers of these factors. Who notices the changes first?	Call the crisis team if after-hours and arrange an urgent assessment if I feel that things are becoming problematical.
If Colin isolates or starts to wonder if people on the street are talking about him or if he generally feels 'paranoid', he is likely to be deteriorating. If he starts to check for cameras and tape recorders, thinks that the TV is talking to him or has active thoughts of becoming violent, these are more serious early warning signs. Reciting prayers is an indication that he is psychotic.	I understand that my case manager may be concerned about my paranoia and worry about me being violent.

WHAT EXTERNAL, ENVIRONMENTAL OR SITUATIONAL FACTORS AFFECT THE RISK? For example, substance use, living conditions, relationship problems, not taking medication etc.	WHAT INTERVENTIONS HELP ADDRESS THESE FACTORS? For example, respite, reducing drug use, phoning a friend.
Colin smoked cannabis until recently. If he restarts, this is likely to increase the risk. He also recently changed his accommodation and is not fully settled yet. He has recently started taking medication but if he stops this, the risk of violence will be increased.	If Colin stops his medication, this should lead to an immediate review of his treatment direction.

WHAT SKILLS OR RESOURCES ARE THE PROTECTIVE FACTORS? For example, insight into illness, supportive family, stable accommodation, compliance with medication etc.	WHO ELSE IS INVOLVED IN THE CARE AND TREATMENT OF THIS PATIENT? Family, friends etc.
Colin has some insight that cannabis abuse is problematical. He has recently stopped his cannabis use. He has not been violent since he was 24 and really wants to stay out of prison.	Colin lives on his own and has few friends.

Have you put enough information in this form to help a colleague treat and care for this patient in an emergency?

Exercise 2 — Monique (continued)

RISK ASSESSMENT AND MANAGEMENT FORM			
DATE OF PLAN	*25 May 2010*	**NAME OF PATIENT**	Place label here
REVIEW DATE (maximum— 6 months)	*25 August 2010*	Surname:	Given name: *Monique*
		DOB:	Patient ID number:

CURRENT DIAGNOSES AND CLINICAL CONCERNS
Include personality traits/disorder.

Monique suffers from schizophrenia with both negative and positive symptoms. She recently broke up with her boyfriend which has distressed her. She continues to smoke marijuana.

CURRENT RISKS
What is/are the risk/s? Who is the risk to, what means might be used and where might it happen?

Monique has risks of relapse of her schizophrenia, suicide when her schizophrenia is uncontrolled and also after major life events.

PREVIOUS EPISODES OF THE RISK(S) Where did it happen, to whom and when? What was the context — illness, situational factors, substance use, not taking medications? Document each episode in as much detail as possible. Identify recurring patterns (risk scenarios) from this information.

When Monique becomes ill, her 'voices' often tell her to kill herself. She has made 3 serious attempts on her life by taking overdoses. The first occurred 5 years ago and the most recent 18 months ago.

Identify early warning signs and triggers of these factors.
Triggers for each overdose have been a relapse of her illness. Early warning signs are poor self-care, preoccupation with voices and upsetting events.

WHAT ARE THE FUNCTIONS OF THE RISK BEHAVIOURS? For example, acting on delusions or hallucinations; self-harm reducing tension or distress, violence or threats being effective, etc.	**WHAT INTERVENTIONS HELP ADDRESS THESE FACTORS? WHAT SKILLS ARE BEING DEVELOPED TO DO THIS?** For example, reality orientation, self-soothing, cognitive skills, DBT skills, etc.
Monique's capacity to ignore the 'voices' becomes less as her mental state deteriorates. She tends to act on the voices to stop them tormenting her and also because she tends to believe them when they say she must die.	If she remembers, sometimes Monique can use the 'reality orientation' techniques she has been taught by her psychologist. These prompt her to question the reality of her 'voices'.

WHAT IN THIS PERSON'S HISTORY CONTRIBUTES TO INCREASING RISK?
For example, substance use, conduct disorder, impulsivity etc. Use the validated scales from your training manual.

Her chronic cannabis use makes it more difficult to control her schizophrenia.

WHAT MENTAL STATE FACTORS INCREASE THESE RISKS? For example, hallucinations, delusions, feelings of rejection, depression etc.	**WHAT INTERVENTIONS HELP ADDRESS THESE FACTORS?** For example, compliance with medication, reduced stress etc.
Monique is more vulnerable at times of major stress. Her hallucinations become more intense and frequent and her capacity to resist them is less. Monique is more at risk of suicide when her symptoms are more intense.	Monique often responds to a brief day in crisis respite. The day hospital can also be used. Monique should be encouraged to stop smoking cannabis but this is difficult for her to do.
Identify early warning signs and triggers of these factors. Who notices the changes first?	
Monique becomes more withdrawn and isolated. She tends to smoke more cannabis, which makes matters worse. Sometimes, Monique starts singing very loudly or shouting at her voices. This is an indication that she is becoming ill.	
WHAT EXTERNAL, ENVIRONMENTAL OR SITUATIONAL FACTORS AFFECT THE RISK? For example, substance use, living conditions, relationship problems, not taking medication etc.	**WHAT INTERVENTIONS HELP ADDRESS THESE FACTORS?** For example, respite, reducing drug use, phoning a friend.
Monique continues to smoke cannabis and says that it helped her cope with the voices. Monique is very vulnerable to rejection. The inpatient environment is a 'safe' place for Monique. She tends to be at low risk when on the ward. Having access to more than 3 days medication is a temptation for Monique to take an overdose.	Using crisis respite and the day hospital often helps Monique reduce her cannabis use. When her symptoms lessen, she is able to reduce her cannabis use herself. When Monique feels rejected, she should be encouraged to look at her cognitive strategies which are in her treatment plan. Medication should be dispensed daily.
WHAT SKILLS OR RESOURCES ARE THE PROTECTIVE FACTORS? For example, insight into illness, supportive family, stable accommodation, compliance with medication etc.	**WHO ELSE IS INVOLVED IN THE CARE AND TREATMENT OF THIS PATIENT?** Family, friends etc.

Monique's mother is supportive. The support staff are clearly concerned about Monique.	Monique has the involvement of the community mental health team including her case manager, psychiatrist and psychologist. The staff at the supported accommodation house all like Monique and her mother is involved by visiting Monique weekly.	
SIGN and PRINT NAME and DESIGNATION	**Date**	**Time**
COMPULSORY COPY TO: Crisis Team and Mental Health Line		
Have you put enough information in this form to help a colleague treat and care for this patient in an emergency?		

Chapter 15
Exercise 1 — identifying personal signals for danger

This is not an unusual scenario. From a personal perspective it is a central task of working in a mental health service to explore personal triggers which may indicate the potential for violence. These will change with your age, your experience and your individual responses to patients. Some clinicians will be triggered by the intense eye contact, some by the patient hitting the wall and some by the memory of the violent incident on the ward 3 months ago. This awareness may also be an opportunity to consider any heuristic biases which may be present (see Chapter 10, page 90). As you become aware of the triggers, you will be able to pick up the early warning signs sooner and the risk of violence towards yourself and other members of your team should lessen. Being able to share your concerns in an environment where staff respect each other and are willing to explore interpersonal feelings is an indication of a healthy working environment.

This is an exercise which should be repeated on a regular basis throughout your career in mental health services. Whenever you have felt threatened or whenever you see a colleague being threatened, it should automatically lead to a review of the context, the patient's mental state and your own responses to this situation. If your team does not facilitate these types of discussions, take the issue to your supervisor or your peer review group. If you have not been in dangerous situations yet, ask your colleagues how they identify their own personal signals. Clinicians often talk about having a gut feeling that something is going to happen. Exploring the gut feeling as much as possible is the task here. Working in an environment in which there are reviews after critical incidents will also help in this process.

Chapter 16

Exercise 1 — Sonny

Over a period of time, you will want to find out the nature of Sonny's previous relationships, how they ended and what allowed them to be sustained. Having a good knowledge of his developmental history, especially his relationship with his mother, will be essential. Depending on your gender, the transference and counter-transferential feelings may also be of use in helping develop an understanding of the meaning of why Sonny only assaults women.

- Do male staff find themselves getting angry with Sonny or possibly having no strong feelings or even an absence of feelings towards him?
- Are female staff fearful because Sonny intrudes upon their personal space or do they find him both charming and threatening, etc?

Discussing your findings with other members of the team will help you develop a more complete understanding of the risk behaviour. With this knowledge, the treatment team should have a greater capacity to predict the situations in which further assaults are more likely to happen.

Exercise 2 — Julie

As with any patient with BPD, being aware of the transference and your counter-transference is vital. Patients with this illness generate powerful emotional responses in others, which can be used to help understand their problems. These patients are often intuitive and will pick up on clinicians' emotions very easily, even if the clinician is trying to hide their feelings. Understanding the meaning of Julie's self-harming behaviour and also the meaning of the interaction between Julie and other members of her family will be essential in the development of a formulation and later a treatment plan. Do the family rescue or reject or both? What is the response of the clinicians?

Exercise 3 — Harry (scapegoating?)

It is unlikely that you will be able to completely manage the situation within the MDT. One solution may be to postpone a decision about Harry and make a time to sit down with the consultant to discuss the consultant's concerns about the use of clozapine. Resolving this problem may lead to a greater capacity to discuss in the MDT the difficulties for the patient without anxiety interfering with the discussion.

Another response may be to use a risk/benefit analysis within the MDT to explore the anxiety experienced by various staff members. It may be more useful to do this in the next MDT once the discussion with the consultant has taken place.

This type of intervention is likely to lead to a review of the risk assessment, which is always a useful undertaking.

Exercise 4 — boundary issues: John, Sarah and Lynley

These patient examples cover the most common counter-transferential issues of rescuing, rejecting and being angry or falling in love with patients. Are you at risk of rescuing or rejecting the patient? How do you manage anger from patients or their relatives? From a risk management perspective, the importance of taking a moment to consider your own feelings and responses cannot be understated. These issues are central to the practice of psychotherapy but are also relevant to everyday practice. Creating your own working environment which provides you with the opportunities to be reflective is an important risk management tool.

Proactive management of these issues is basically the same as the management of personal responses to risk as described on page 46. Reflection, supervision and good peer discussions will go a long way towards managing these potential problems. Having a team leader who facilitates these discussions is invaluable. Good protocols, policies and guidelines help provide boundaries for clinicians to work within.

For those clinicians who repeatedly struggle with these issues, consideration should be given to personal psychotherapy to reduce the risk of infecting interpersonal relationships with their own difficulties.

▇▌ GLOSSARY

Affect storms: A reaction triggered by intense anxiety. They occur when there are threats to defensive structures (e.g. a persona designed to protect against deep-seated feelings of worthlessness) and are characterised by explosions of emotional expression which cannot be modulated by a patient or modified easily by clinical intervention.

Catastrophise: An irrational thought that something is far worse than it actually is.

Causal risk factor: A risk factor that can be changed by manipulation and when changed can be shown to alter the risk.

Cognitive dissonance: An uncomfortable feeling caused by holding two contradictory ideas simultaneously.

Compassion fatigue: *see* vicarious traumatisation.

Counter-transference: A redirection of a therapist's feelings toward a client, or more generally a therapist's emotional entanglement with a client. A therapist's attunement to his or her own counter-transference is nearly as critical as his or her understanding of the transference.

Dissociation: A perceived detachment of the mind from the emotional state or even from the body. Dissociation is characterised by a sense of the world as a dreamlike or unreal place and may be accompanied by poor memory of the specific events, which in severe form is known as 'dissociative amnesia'.

Heuristics: Cognitive shortcuts that allow decisions to be made in conditions of uncertainty.

Level of risk: = Likelihood + Consequences of the outcome.

Likelihood: = Contextual factors × Patient risk factors.

Mentalisation: The ability to understand oneself by inferring the mental states that lie behind overt behaviour.

Persecutory ideation: Thoughts and/or sense of being persecuted by others.

Repetition compulsion: Repetition compulsion is a psychological phenomenon in which a person repeats a traumatic event or its circumstances over and over again. This includes re-enacting the event or putting oneself in situations that have a high probability of the event occurring again.

Risk: The likelihood of an adverse event or outcome. The possibility of incurring misfortune or loss.

Risk acceptance: An informed decision to accept the consequences and likelihood of a particular risk.

Risk assessment: The overall process of risk analysis and weighing up the risk.

Risk evaluation (weighing up the risk): The process used to determine risk management priorities, often by using a risk/benefit analysis.

Risk factor: Something in the patient's history or current environment or mental state which makes the risk more likely to occur.

Risk identification: The process of determining what can happen, why and how.

Risk level: The level of risk calculated as a function of likelihood and consequences.

Risk management: The culture, processes and structures that are directed towards the effective management of risks and potential opportunities.

Risk mitigation: Mitigating the consequences of risk outcomes should they occur.

Risk state: The synthesis of the static and dynamic risk factors.

Secondary PTSD: *see* vicarious traumatisation.

Secondary risk management: Clinicians making management decisions to reduce their own anxiety and not focussing on the needs of the patient.

Stakeholders: Those people and organisations who may affect, be affected by, or perceive themselves to be affected by, the decisions or activities of the service.

Transference: A reproduction of emotions relating to repressed experiences, especially of childhood, and the substitution of another person for the original object of the repressed impulses.

Vicarious traumatisation: This is sometimes called secondary PTSD or compassion fatigue. It is a process whereby a person (usually a clinician) either witnessing traumatic episodes or listening to trauma stories develops symptomatology of, or behaviors similar to, PTSD.

INDEX